My
Myasthenia Gravis

STEPHEN LAU

This book is dedicated to those,
who are afflicted with myasthenia gravis,
or any autoimmune disease,
as well as those who adopt a holistic approach
to enhance their health and wellbeing.

STEPHEN LAU

CONTENTS

FOREWORD

Most probably you bought this book because you have been diagnosed with an autoimmune disease, or your loved one has developed an autoimmune disorder, such as *myasthenia gravis* or rheumatoid arthritis. It is my wish that you find the content of this book informative and useful in helping you or your loved one improve the autoimmune disease conditions and symptoms.

The content is intended for general information purpose only, and therefore does not constitute any medical advice. As a matter of fact, this book is not intended to be a source of *any* advice, and thus you should not rely on any information provided in the book as such.

This book is about "my" *myasthenia gravis*: how I got the disorder, how I struggled with its many symptoms, and how I have successfully overcome many of its symptoms. This is the second edition: I have updated some of the information and included more; hopefully, this new input will help you in the lifelong journey to coping with this "incurable" disease.

Now, as I look back, I think getting my *myasthenia gravis* was a blessing in disguise. Everything happens in one's life with a divine purpose. In a way, I was grateful that I *had* the illness—which has changed my life forever and for the better. For one thing, without my *myasthenia gravis*, I would not have written this book, and many other books on health and healing. For another, my *myasthenia gravis* was a self-awakening for me. Oftentimes in life, it would take a crisis, such as a disease, for self-enlightenment. My *myasthenia gravis* was a wakeup call for me: it not only initiated my passionate pursuit of health and healing in my life but also enlightened me with the wisdom in living, which plays a pivotal part in my golden years. To me, my *myasthenia gravis* was indeed a blessing in disguise—a misfortune that I have to be thankful for.

It is important that you willingly accept your fate of getting the autoimmune disorder as the first step in your battle against *myasthenia gravis*. It is futile to ask the question: *Why me?* Embracing whatever that comes along in your life, no matter what, is life transformation. I did not blame anyone or anything for my illness, nor did I have any regret. I totally accepted my fate.

Recognition and acceptance of one's conditions is the first positive step towards natural self-healing. Denial and despair, on the other hand, would only put more roadblocks to self-healing and recovery. I was determined to find out the *causes* of my health problems. I wanted to know *why* I was struck down with *myasthenia gravis*. With that intent, I began to empower myself with knowledge to deal with the disease itself and cope with its many symptoms.

I hope you enjoy reading this book, and wish you all the best in your recovery and recuperation!

Stephen Lau
Copyright© by Stephen Lau

INTRODUCTION

Myasthenia gravis is only one of the many autoimmune diseases that affect humans, and there are over one hundred of them.

The Immune System

"In recent years science has learned that the human immune system is much more complicated than we thought." **Dr. Philip F. Incao**, M.D.

First and foremost, you must have an understanding of your immune system in simple layman's terms:

Antibodies are proteins that protect the human body from disease and disorder, and they are like soldiers in an army.

Antigens are foreign invaders in the form of bacteria and viruses that attack the human body.

T-cells, a type of white blood cells originating from the bone marrow, either control and regulate the immune response or directly attack infected cells.

The human immune system is complicated in that it affects the *whole* body system in many different ways. As such, it can heal you but it can also harm you. It protects your cells and maintains your overall health through its production of antibodies (specific proteins) to fight against antigens (invaders to your body system). However, an impaired or dysfunctional immune system can adversely affect your overall health because it is the common denominator of more than one hundred autoimmune diseases.

The immune system is basically made up of four parts, and each part has its unique functions; it involves the whole human body, not just certain body organs and tissues. The complexity of the human immune system is a testament to the ingenuity and mystery of human creation.

The basic function of the immune system is to warn the body of imminent dangers of viruses and bacteria (unfortunately, many of us just ignore these tale-telling signs, or simply fail to decipher these subtle body messages warning us of an imminent disease). In addition, the immune system "remembers" these foreign invaders or antigens (the intention is to identify similar invaders in future for better disease-prevention purpose). Furthermore, the white blood cells in the immune system produce antibodies, which are chemicals that attach to and attack specific antigens. These white blood cells also send "messages" that will cause "inflammation" in response to an injury or antigen, and thus instrumental in preventing an infection from spreading elsewhere. In other words, they receive "chemical instructions" to nip the disease or infection in the bud.

In short, the immune system serves different functions of *identification*, *activation*, *mobilization*, and *restoration*. It is akin to a police department in a city: it recognizes the city's potential crime scenario, takes strong measures to protect the public, trains the local police force to take appropriate action, and regulates the law and order of the city.

Autoimmune Diseases

An autoimmune disease is a result of the breakdown or malfunction of the immune system. There are more than one hundred immune disorders and diseases.

The immune attack can target any area, such as the joints, causing rheumatoid arthritis, the thyroid gland, leading to an overactive or underactive thyroid, and nerve cells, resulting in multiple sclerosis, among others. Very often, the immune attack may have several targets; that is, if you have one autoimmune disease, you are at risk for a second or even a third disease, especially if you have not taken good care of your immune system. In addition, an attack may have remission, followed by worsening of symptoms. Therefore, the battle against an autoimmune disease is not only challenging, but also devastating.

Autoimmune diseases are becoming more rampant. By and large, women are more vulnerable to them than men are. Men have a higher incidence of mellitus diabetes and myocarditis (inflammation of the heart) than women; other than those, women are 3 to 6 times more prone to autoimmune diseases than their opposite sex.

Modern medicine is unable to explain or specifically identify the underlying causes of autoimmune diseases. Despite the advancement of modern science and technology, frustration and disappointment are part of modern medicine in the area of immune dysfunction. Without the capability to identify the causes of autoimmune diseases, there is no cure to date. Accordingly, modern medicine focuses on addressing the symptoms rather than the causes.

The Alternatives

In the past two decades or so, many have sought medical treatments for their "incurable" diseases, using herbs, detoxification, homeopathy, vitamins, and minerals. This holistic non-drug approach to disease control and elimination has come to be known as alternative medicine.

Nowadays, medical universities in the United States, as well as in other parts of the world, are offering alternative medicine courses and complementary medicine programs, while research studies on plant nutrients and vitamins and minerals are being conducted in university laboratories and clinical settings. They are all strong testaments to the effectiveness of alternative disease treatments.

Indeed, in this day and age, many people are becoming frustrated with conventional medicine's drugs, and the cut-and-burn approaches to disease. However, if you wish to seek an alternative approach to drug therapies, you should first educate yourself by reading books and other relevant materials. It is critically important to empower yourself with knowledge *before* you make any medical decision. But the decision should be totally *yours*, because nobody knows better than yourself the health conditions of your own body.

<u>ONE</u>

THE AUTOIMMUNITY ATTACK

Autoimmunity

Autoimmunity occurs when the immune system attacks its own cells, "mistaking" them for foreign invaders.

The healthy human body is equipped with immunity to fight against viruses, bacteria, and parasites—in short, diseases. Unfortunately, this immunity provider, known as the immune system, may become compromised or dysfunctional such that, instead of attacking the unwelcome foreign invaders to the body, it begins to attack the cells and tissues within the body itself.

In a healthy individual, the immune defenses protect the cells from outside invaders, but when a person develops autoimmunity, the immune system mistakenly attacks the body's own cells instead of protecting them. To illustrate, in *myasthenia gravis*, which is an autoimmune disease, it is an autoantibody attack on the receptor responsible for the communication between the nervous system and voluntary muscles, and thus causing some miscommunication that may result in muscle weakness, or not responding appropriately, which is one of the hallmark characteristics of *myasthenia gravis.*

Autoimmune Disorders

The good news is that autoimmunity is present in everyone to some extent. The bad news is that autoimmunity can be triggered by many environmental, physical, as well as emotional factors, such that it can cause a broad spectrum of human illnesses, known as autoimmune diseases, which, according to modern Western medicine, has no known cure.

Essentially, autoimmunity can affect almost *any* organ or body system. The exact problem you may have with autoimmunity depends on which body tissues are being targeted by your immune system. For example, if your skin is targeted, you may have skin rashes, blisters, or color changes; if your thyroid gland is affected, you may feel extremely tired, sensitive to cold, and muscle aches; if your joints are attacked, you may have severe joint pain, stiffness, and loss of joint function.

There are more than 100 types of autoimmune diseases, including *multiple sclerosis, type 1 diabetes mellitus, rheumatoid arthritis,* and *myasthenia gravis,* among many others.

The Potential Causes

This concept of autoimmunity as the cause of human illness is relatively new, and it was accepted into the mainstream medicine only about half a century ago. At present, the medical community is still very much at a loss as to *how* autoimmunity develops in an individual, although now there is increasing evidence linking environmental agents to autoimmune diseases. These may include infectious agents, such as viruses, pharmaceutical and chemical agents, heavy metals, dietary factors, including food allergies, as well as a number of biological agents, such as genetic disposition. However, medical scientists are still unable to pinpoint the exact cause of autoimmune diseases. As a result, many new experimental drugs have been developed to treat autoimmunity. Unfortunately, many of these experimental drugs may also be toxic to the body with long-term adverse side effects on the patient's health.

The Risk Factors

The age factor

The immune system becomes less effective as aging continues. Therefore, the elderly are more susceptible to developing autoimmune diseases. However, it must be pointed out that autoimmune diseases do develop in the adult population as early as in the twenties and thirties.

The gender factor

Most autoimmune diseases strike women more than they do men, particularly women of working age and during their child-bearing years.

The genetic factor

The inherited genes may predispose an individual to developing an autoimmune disease.

The stress factor

Excess stress may trigger the onset of an autoimmune

disease in an individual already with an over-stressed or a weakened immune system. Stress is the major factor in most human diseases.

The virus factor

An individual vulnerable to virus infections is also at risk for developing an autoimmune disease.

The Cellular Health

Cells make up your organs. When your cells die, your organs fail and health deteriorates; as a result, you age and die.

To maintain and sustain life, some of your cells replicate themselves continually, such as epithelial cells in your intestine, while others do not divide, such as your heart cells and neurons in your brain.

The good news is that, on average, most normal human cells have more than 100 years of lifespan built into them.

The bad news is that all human cells require *energy* and *oxygen* to function normally, and in this oxidative process *free radicals* are created. For example, when you breathe in life-giving oxygen, you also breathe out harmful carbon dioxide. This oxidative process is how your Creator has ingeniously built normal cell death into your body system to ensure your mortality. Slowly and accumulatively, these free radicals build up in your cells, leading to premature cell death. You cannot prolong your life indefinitely, but you can extend your lifespan by slowing down the oxidative process of free radicals. In other words, eradication of free radicals holds the key to optimum health and longevity.

Premature cell death is due to both human and environmental factors, such as bacteria and viruses, free radicals, toxins, and trauma, which can cause irreparable damage to your cells, and thus instrumental in accelerating the demise of these cells. However, many of these factors are not only avoidable but also preventable.

Essentially, genes play an important role in determining the quality of your cells. In other words, your genetic time clock governs how long your cells will live and survive. Your main objective is to *outpace* your genetic time clock. Remember, nothing is set in stone; you always have a choice—the choice is all yours.

The Damage of Body Cells

Your body is composed of negatively and positively charged molecules, which must be balanced in order to enable your cells to function normally. A free radical is formed when there is *imbalance* in these molecules. A free radical also damages other molecules, causing them to produce more free radicals—and thus creating a chain reaction of damages that become the scourges of aging and the sources of disease and disorders, in particular, autoimmune diseases.

The damages by free radicals

There are several types of free radicals, and oxygen free radicals are most damaging, especially to your DNA and cell membranes.

Your cells require oxygen for survival. Unfortunately, what gives life also takes away life. In the process of oxidation, harmful oxygen free radicals are produced. Oxygen free radicals and other free radicals in your body cause damages to your cells.

Brain damage

The neurons in your brain may also become damaged by free radicals. The damage may be irreparable because the neurons, unlike other cells, cannot replicate themselves.

Cellular damage

The cumulative damage to your DNA by free radicals is a major contributing factor to many autoimmune diseases, including human cancers.

Heart damage

When your LDL or "bad cholesterol" is attacked by free radicals, they become more attached to the walls of your arteries, and thus forming plagues to block the free flow of blood to your heart.

The only way to fight against free radicals is by boosting your body's own immunity.

Boosting Immunity

As you age, your immune system becomes weaker, as evidenced by the high incidence of influenza and pneumonia after age 25, not to mention among the elderly. Therefore, it is very important to boost your immunity, which is closely related to your thymus (the commander-in-chief of fighters in your immune system against foreign invaders), with the 10 most important nutritional supplements:

- Vitamin A to prevent thymus shrinkage (5,000 IU

daily dosage)

- Vitamin B_6 to maintain hormone lev᷏ prevent thymus shrinkage (50 mg daily do᷏ ᷏ ᷏)

- Vitamin C to regulate T-cell (white blood thymus cells) function (at least 1,000 mg daily dosage or up to bowel tolerance)

- Vitamin E to increase infection resistance (400 - 800 IU daily dosage)

- Selenium to increase T-cell activity and antibody production for detoxification (100 mcg daily dosage)

- Zinc to boost your thymus for maturing T-cells to fight invaders (15 mg daily dosage)

- Coenzyme CO_{10} to increase energy production for cells' activities

- L-glutathione to regenerate immune cells in the immune system (200 mg daily dosage)

- Magnesium to increase enzymatic reactions (100 mg daily dosage)

- DHEA to control cortisol, the stress hormone (5 mg daily dosage)

Protecting the Immune System

In addition to taking nutritional supplements to boost your immunity, you need to use *diet*, such as a natural hyroid diet, to protect your immune system.

Eat fresh, organic fruits, vegetables, seeds and nuts daily.

Eating Natural Foods

Eat raw occasionally. Cooking, food processing, and freezing destroy some of the health-promoting nutrients, such as enzymes, in your foods.

Eat phytonutrients, which are plant nutrients. These powerful nutrients include carotenoids, flavonoids, and phytosterols, among others.

Carotenoids

Dark green, yellow, red, and orange vegetables and fruits are rich in carotenoids. These potent antioxidants against free radicals include the following: bilberries, blueberries, broccoli, carrots, citrus fruits, ginkgo biloba, grapes, green tea, onions, peppers, and tangerines.

Phytosterols

Phytosterols are plant fats (just like animal fats). Plant fats inhibit the secretion of inflammatory cytokines (pain-causing agents), and are effective in controlling rheumatoid arthritis, one of the most debilitating and difficult-to-treat autoimmune diseases today.

Foods rich in phytosterols include the following: almonds, cashews, sesame seeds, sunflower seeds, barley, peas, and soybeans.

However, your body may have difficulty in absorbing plant fats, and therefore take a supplement of sterinol daily.

TWO

MY STORY

Myasthenia Gravis

Myasthenia gravis is an autoimmune neuromuscular disease characterized by varying degrees of weakness and fatigue of the skeletal (voluntary) muscles of the body. This muscular dysfunctional condition is believed to result from an immune disorder that causes the neurotransmitter *acetylcholine* to become less effective. Some muscle groups, such as the eye muscles, the face and throat muscles, and muscles in the arms and legs, are more commonly and easily affected by this neurotransmitter.

Essentially, the hallmark of the disease is muscle weakness, which increases during periods of activity and improves after periods of rest. Muscle weakness may adversely affect the way of life, such as vision, (muscles that control eye and eyelid movements), facial expression (facial muscles), breathing, talking, chewing and swallowing (neck and throat muscles), and body movements.

Myasthenia gravis is more common in women younger

than 40 and in men older than 60.

My Story

Many years ago, I was afflicted with *myasthenia gravis*. I was undergoing a most stressful episode in my life. I was in my fifties—call it midlife crisis if you would. One day I felt intense pressure on my eyes. My first concern was glaucoma (a condition of increased fluid pressure inside the eye).

Immediately, I went to see an ophthalmologist, who subsequently referred me to a neurologist, who was. at that time the head of the neurology department in a well-known healthcare system in Cleveland, Ohio. After running some medical tests, he confirmed his diagnosis that I had *myasthenia gravis*.

My Conditions

I had developed ocular symptoms: ptosis (drooping of eyelids) and diplopia (double vision) in my *myasthenia gravis*.

My neck and limb muscles were also weak. I had to use a neck-rest to prop up my head when I drove; I could hardly use my fingers to control the mouse when I used my computer; and I could not raise my left hand without using my right hand to help prop it up.

Fortunately, I did not experience any weakness of the muscles of my pharynx, which could cause difficulty in chewing and swallowing, as well as slurred speech, in many cases of *myasthenia gravis*.

Naturally, I was devastated at the diagnosis and the conditions of my *myasthenia gravis*, which all happened within a matter of days. Worst of all, the neurologist told me that there was no known cure, although he reassured me that he could improve my disease symptoms.

Deep down, I knew it was stress that triggered the onset of my *myasthenia gravis*, but it was by no means the only cause. I also knew that if I did not have it then, I would probably have it further down the road. It was just a matter of time—only at that time I was not aware that I had been having the problem all along. I was carrying a ticking time-bomb too ready to explode on me.

Initially, I was confused and befuddled: *Why* did I get sick? For the past several decades, my health had been good, if not excellent—or so I thought. All those years prior to my *myasthenia gravis*, I had been quite health conscious in matters of foods and drinks; I had never been hospitalized all my life, and before the onset of my myasthenia gravis, I seldom paid a visit to the doctor. I had been having a clean bill of health up until then.

So, what was wrong with me?

I began to do some soul-searching and looked into my past.

Unlike most other kids, I did not have chicken pox until I was a teenager. That was a tale-telling sign that my immune system was *different* from that of others, or at least not as good as I thought it was. There was something amiss, but I did not know exactly what it was and I could not put a finger on it.

Then I recalled that when I was a child, I had been constantly bed-ridden with fever and coughing—my mother always worried that I could get infections from other kids, or worse, I would not live long.

I remember I never liked green vegetables and fish—which I would gobble up, stuff them in my mouth, and then spit them out as soon as I got out of the house. That was how bad I was!

As I stepped into my teens, my health conditions

suddenly and significantly improved. In fact, all my symptoms of ill health disappeared soon after I had my chicken pox at the age of thirteen or fourteen. The experience of my chicken pox was excruciating, but it seemed to have changed my health conditions completely for the better.

Ever since then, I had not had any major physical ailment, except that I was still susceptible to the common cold—which I often overdosed myself with over-the-counter cold medications. I did not know that all those years I had been shuffling chemical toxins into my body!

There was another episode during my young adulthood. I was frequently involved in some artwork, which required me to make some fiberglass from newspapers by pouring some chemical solution over them. On one occasion, I accidentally mixed some toxic chemicals, giving out some toxic fume. After inhaling it, I passed out for some minutes, and I felt sick for several days.

My regular exposure to toxic chemicals in my artwork through inhalation must have damaged my immune system. Maybe the damage done was long-term and irreparable.

Nevertheless, for many decades, I had enjoyed relatively good health—or so I thought.

In my late forties, I had shingles—which was another red flag that there was something wrong with my immune system. However, I did not pay much attention to that episode that lasted several days.

In my early fifties, the stress in my life eventually triggered the onset of my *myasthenia gravis*, which was the outcome of my over-stressed immune system.

My Treatment

At first, I was prescribed *pyridostigmine* (*mestinon*) as the usual first-line treatment for my *myasthenia gravis*.

After several months, my conditions did not improve much. I was given another prescription, *prednisone*, a synthetic hormone commonly referred to as a "steroid," for my myasthenia gravis. *Prednisone* acts as long-term immunosuppressant to suppress the production of antibodies. Essentially, it serves to stabilize my so-called "overactive" immune system.

The adverse side effects of *prednisone* for my myasthenia gravis included my decreased resistance to infection, indigestion, hypertension, weight gain, swelling of the face, thinning of skin, predisposition to osteoporosis, and potential development of cataracts and glaucoma.

The long list was not only depressing but also frightening. I was worried that I would have to take all my medications for the rest of my life not just for my *myasthenia gravis* but also for the many side effects of those medications for *myasthenia graves*, such as bone loss, weight gain, and high blood pressure, among others.

In the beginning, there was some improvement in the symptoms, but overall most of the symptoms were still there, and I was never lucky enough to experience some remission from the disease symptoms.

After almost two years on *prednisone*, my neurologist, seeing that there was little improvement in my *myasthenia gravis*, switched me to *azathioprine*, supposedly with fewer side effects. That medication did not seem to have any significant effect on my symptoms.

My Rude Awakening

I was in a dilemma: on the one hand, I needed improvement in my neuromuscular transmission to increase my muscle strength and eliminate my double vision; on the other hand, I knew that if *myasthenia gravis* did not kill me, the many side effects of the medications eventually would.

Then I made a decision to change drastically my diet in an attempt to discontinue my medications ultimately. The initial results were quite encouraging: I began to experience some improvement in my symptoms. Instead of gaining weight, I lost a few pounds; instead of jacking up my blood pressure, I made it plummet. I had won my first battle against the initial adverse side effects of medications of *myasthenia gravis*.

I knew that I had to do more—much more than that. I was in for my rude awakening: there was no miracle cure for my *myasthenia gravis*; only my holistic wellness would bring about recovery and natural healing.

The Road to Self-Healing

For me, the road to recovery had been a long and winding one.

I recognized that my immune system is not only an integrated network of cells that would protect me in times of an infection, but also a system with its many regulatory mechanisms that, if uncontrolled, would become my enemy instead of my friend.

I also realized that my immune system has to be protected by being fed the correct foods, as well as being given the optimum environment free from physical, emotional, and psychological stress, which may affect my immune system negatively.

Most important of all, I understood that my wholesome well-being, unlike my medications that "switched" off my immuno-response when it was overactive, may hold the key to my ultimate recovery and recuperation.

My parents might not have given me an excellent immune system. I could not have chosen my parents, but I can certainly choose *my* lifestyle, and I can control what I put into my body and even what comes out of my body.

I was determined to take matters into my own hands. I had to control my own health destiny.

I cherished the strong conviction that whatever my mind can conceive and believe I can achieve.

Meanwhile, I was also fully aware of the overpowering forces of Nature. To combat Nature is futile, but I can command Nature by *obeying* it, instead of going *against* it.

> "Like water, soft and yielding,
> yet it overcomes the hard and the rigid.
> Stiffness and stubbornness cause much suffering.
> We all intuitively know
> that flexibility and tenderness are the way to go.
> Yet our conditioned minds
> tell us to go the other way."
> (**Lao Tzu**, *Tao Te Ching*, Chapter 78)

To obey Nature involves the recognition of the natural self-healing power of my physical body—if given the *right* environment.

The right environment implies that my body must be *clean* enough internally.

Initially, I had attempted several 24-hour fasts. Finally, I decided to take the plunge: a longer fast for more than three weeks, during which I consumed no solid food, except plain water.

It was a miracle to me.

Surprisingly, I did not feel any physical weakness, not to mention any pangs of hunger. I lost some fifteen pounds. I was not overweight prior to the fast, so people were wondering if I was sick. I told them I had to cleanse myself so that I would not be sick again. Most of them did not have a clue as to what I was saying, and responded, "If you don't want to be sick, you should eat *more*, not less! Stephen, you look too thin, and not healthy at all." How could a fish explain to a bird what water is like!

The internal cleansing initiated by the longer fast set the groundwork for my subsequent lifestyle changes. I was well on the road to self-healing.

Slowly and gradually, I reduced my medications, until I stopped *all* medications, and I even stopped seeing my doctor—that happened within three to four months.

That was almost two decades ago. Now, I am in my early seventies: my blood pressure and cholesterol numbers are all normal; I am not overweight. Above all, as of now, I am not taking ANY medication at all, as opposed to taking more than ten medications a day nearly two decades ago.

You, too, can enjoy good health, which is man's greatest asset, if you just go on reading the rest of my book.

THREE

UNDERSTANDING SELF-HEALING

The Miracle of Self-Healing

Albert Einstein once said: "There are two ways to live: you can live as if nothing is a miracle; you can live as if everything is a miracle." So, believe in self-healing, and live your life as if everything is a miracle—including the miracle to heal yourself of *myasthenia gravis*. Yes, self-healing is a miracle of life.

Ironically enough, modern Western medicine has led many of us to believe that healing is a complex process, involving high technology, complex drugs, and state-of-the-art procedures. It is human nature to learn belief systems, theories, and facts without challenging them. Truly, medical professionals are experts in their respective fields, and, obviously, they not only know more than we do but also have more experience than we have. However, that does not imply that we should readily accept *all* their opinions without fully understanding what they are. Unfortunately, many of us are doing just *that*—going along with what they say, despite the many mistakes, even many fatal ones, made by these professionals. As a matter of fact, according to a study in the *Journal of the American Medical Association*, more than 100,000 Americans died in hospitals from dangerous drugs or from their dangerous side effects in 1998.

To make the miracle of self-healing a reality for your autoimmune disease, understand the essentials of self-healing.

The Essentials of Self-Healing

The Power of the Mind

Healing begins with the mind *first* and not the body.

The mind is powerful in that it is the origin of all your thoughts, which determine not only *who* you are but also *how* you experience your life. Life is a journey of experiences, throughout which the mind plays a pivotal part. Whether an individual is going to be healthy, successful, or happy in life depends on the power of the mind. Mind power is the essence of being. Mind power holds the key to recovery from any disease, including yours from your autoimmune disease. Every thought counts in the process of self-healing.

If you wish to combat, if not to totally cure yourself of, an autoimmune disease, you must first of all have the *intent* to heal, without which there is no self-cure or recovery, and your battle against the autoimmune disease is already half-lost.

With *intent*, come *concentration* and *focus* to seek self-help to empower yourself with knowledge of self-healing, without which you may be at a loss as to what to do next. Out of sheer ignorance, many simply turn to conventional medicine for treatment; unfortunately, it may be a case of jumping from the frying pan into the fire.

Mind power is also evidenced in its capability to create

"reality." Yes, it is all in the mind, and it is always mind over matter.

A powerful mind can produce positive thoughts, which affect not just your body and your emotions, but also your genes.

As a matter of fact, according to scientific studies, how your mind processes your daily experiences can even turn on or off a particular gene responsible for a particular disease. In other words, there is a close body-mind connection with respect to health and healing.

Utilize your mind power to create the "reality" of healing for your autoimmune disease. That is, you need *visualization*, which is the ability to see "reality" in your mind's eye. Seeing is believing: "seeing" the positive result of your efforts through positive images reinforces your "believing" that you will be cured of your *myasthenia gravis* symptoms.

The road to health and recovery from an autoimmune disease is never direct or smooth: it is always paved with roadblocks and detours in the form of relapses and remission. As a result, you will need determination and perseverance before you can reach your goal of self-healing. Given the uniqueness of each individual's physical and physiological makeup, you must use your *imagination* and *creativity* to devise your own methods of self-cure for your *myasthenia gravis*.

Creative visualization is a powerful tool to enhance your mind power for mind healing to initiate the subsequent body healing. That is, *manifestation* of the mind may begin to manifest itself in the body healing process.

The concept of creative visualization has been around for decades.

One of the most important rules for visualization is that it should be done in the present tense. For example, if you desire muscle strength, you should be visualizing yourself free of muscle weakness, and feeling the moment as if it is happening this instant and not some time in the future. In other words, feel the sense of joy of freedom of movement, rather than the sense of wanting or desiring for it. In addition, you must visualize with specific details to authenticate the reality of your visualization. Furthermore, you must be consistent and persistent in your visualization. Remember, your mind is a muscle too: you must exercise it constantly and consistently to create the desirable strength to accomplish its mission.

Is creative visualization no more than a placebo effect?

Placebo effect is not just offering magic, hope, and comfort for a cure of a disease. The truth is that the placebo effect is significant—as much as between 35 and 75 percent of patients benefit from taking a dummy pill in studies of new drugs.

If placebos are lies, they can also be "lies that heal." The placebo effect is not limited to the subjective sensations of patients; some studies have shown actual physiological change as a result of sham treatments. For example, doctors in one study successfully eliminated warts by painting them with a brightly colored, inert dye and reassuring patients that the warts would be gone once the color wore off.

Albert Einstein once said: "Imagination is more important than knowledge." Remember, you imagination is a powerful mental tool to help you achieve your goal in self-healing by vibrating your mental energies in a positive way.

Changing the Subconscious Mind to Heal

The human brain has about 15 billion cells, and you may

have utilized only about 10 to 15 percent of your brain power, so there is still plenty of room for enhancing your mind power. In other words, your brain has great potential power for mind healing.

You can significantly increase your brain power with *practices* and *exercises* to train your brain. Although everyone's brain differs, everyone can empower his or her mind, given the proper tools and training.

The mind—the consciousness of the brain—has two major components: the *conscious* mind, and the *subconscious* mind.

The conscious mind makes decisions, but the subconscious mind directs the conscious mind. That is to say, in your conscious mind, you are fully aware of your own actions and their respective consequences; in your subconscious mind, but in reality you only respond *spontaneously* to repetitions of words and images in the form of affirmation and visualization.

Use positive affirmation to change your subconscious mind, thereby instrumental in changing your conscious mind to begin changing your lifestyle to initiate your self-healing process.

Optimizing Subliminal Messages

The laws of nature determine how things happen. One of the laws of nature is *habitual stimulus*: a certain stimulus, habitually applied time after time, may prove to produce a certain predictable result. Therefore, you can shape your thoughts into definite patterns, and act accordingly through consistency and regularity. In that way, you can *control* what you think in order to *change* your habits, that is, *consciously* changing your thoughts. Unlike animals following only their natural instincts, you have the capability to control your mind by manipulating your thoughts through repetitions of self-suggestions in the form of both words and visual images.

Use subliminal messages to conduct an *internal dialogue* with your subconscious mind in order to achieve your personal goals in life, to enhance your well-being, and to promote your physical and spiritual wellness.

A subliminal message or self-suggestion is an idea or notion that elicits a response in thought or behavior. It can derive from another person, such as a comment or criticism by that person; it can stem from an object, such as a bill requiring some action. A suggestion can, of course, come from *self* in the form of self-talk or self-persuasion, such as when you are telling yourself that it is all right to eat junk food occasionally (which, incidentally, is an example of a negative self-suggestion).

A subliminal message is an effective means to communicate with the inner or subconscious mind, which is powerful in that it not only runs the autonomic functions of your body but also controls your immune system. It can bring about a positive change in your thoughts and thinking through the production of endorphins (the feel-good hormones), thereby either making you positive or inducing negativity, and thus positively or adversely changing your general outlook of life and self.

Life is full of choices, and a self-suggestion can indeed affect your choices, and hence the quality of your life.

For a subliminal message to be effective and powerful, however, it has to be repeated over and over again until the intention is absorbed and registered in the subconscious mind.

Subliminal messages have to be *simple*, *relevant*, and *realistic*. You must strongly believe in the veracity of those messages. In other words, you must be honest with yourself in believing that those subliminal messages are achievable goals in your life. Buying a lottery ticket, for example, and believing that it will ultimately change your life is not a realistic subliminal message.

Given that subliminal messages in the form of words have to be repeated over and over again until their powerful intentions are deeply ingrained and etched in your subconscious mind, *simplicity*, *consistency*, and *persistency* are the characteristics critical to their success.

To illustrate, repeat to yourself daily the following positive affirmations or subliminal messages:

- I am now showing the desire, learning the know-how, and acquiring the skills to change my thoughts in order to change my lifestyle to enhance my immune system.

- I am now willing to accept any change in order to become a healthier individual than I am right now.

- I am now learning how to change my thoughts in order to change my thinking in matters of health and healing.

- I am now changing on the inside to bring about positive changes on the outside.

Subliminal messages in the form of powerful images and symbols are most effective and powerful when your body and mind are in a relaxed state, such as in a deep meditation, during which your mind is free from any five-sense activity.

Mental commitment is mental responsibility, without which nothing can be accomplished. In life, there is no free lunch: you must work at it in order to achieve it. Use your subliminal messages to promote your mental commitment to changing your thinking:

- I am a responsible person and I am totally committed to changing my thoughts.

- I am staying committed until I reach my goal to change my thinking through daily subliminal messages.

- I am committed to empowering my mind with subliminal messages in words and images.

Use positive affirmations or self-suggestions as powerful intents in the subconscious mind instrumental in changing negative thoughts into positive ones in your conscious mind. Meanwhile, reinforce your self-suggestions with powerful visual images. Remember, a picture is worth a thousand words. Visualize the outcomes of your positive affirmations; see yourself healed of your *myasthenia gravis*.

FOUR

STOP ALL DANGEROUS DRUGS

When a healthy individual gets sick, usually the first impulse of that individual is to rush to see a doctor to get the condition "fixed." Unfortunately, modern medicine, despite its enormous advances in the understanding of health and diseases, shows inadequate understanding of the origin and perpetuation of disease. Western medicine emphasizes too much the theoretical framework of disease, while ignoring the workings of the human body itself. Such disproportionate emphasis has led to the undue focus on drugs and surgeries to carry out the task of healing, instead of relying on the body itself.

But everything you do—including what you touch, breathe, eat, and even think—affects your immunity, and hence may become the source of your diseases and disorders. Without taking that into consideration, simply focusing on "fixing" the symptoms will never work.

Ovid, the ancient Roman poet once commented: "Medicine sometimes snatches away health, sometimes gives it." Therefore, medicine can be your friend or your foe. Just beware!

No Cure for Autoimmune Diseases

According to the medical community, there is no known cure for *myasthenia gravis*, or any autoimmune disease, for that matter. That is not surprising, given the complexity of autoimmunity and the approach of conventional medicine to disease treatment. Western medicine uses pharmaceutical drugs to deal with the various symptoms of different types of autoimmune diseases by suppressing the overactive immune system. But an autoimmune disease involves not just the mind, but also many different organs of the body—in fact, the *whole* body or the *personality* of the individual afflicted with an autoimmune disease.

Myasthenia gravis can be so varied and different in each individual that treatment also becomes so highly individualized according to the severity of the disorder, age, sex, as well as the degree of functional impairment. The need for medication may even vary considerably from day to day in response to emotional stress, infections, and even the hot weather.

Mestinon, Regonol, and *Prostigmin* are the most commonly used oral medications to treat muscle weakness without affecting the underlying disease that causes it. Therefore, these drugs are often given in conjunction with other treatments. All these drugs have different side effects: narrowing of the muscle of the iris in the eye, causing the pupil to become smaller; increased nasal and bronchial secretions, as well as increased saliva and urination; loose stools, diarrhea, vomiting, and abdominal cramps; and urinary tract infections, among many other undesirable side effects.

Other possible treatment may include *thymectomy*, which is the removal of the thymus to increase the frequency of *myasthenia gravis* remission.

Corticosteroid drugs, such as *prednisone*, are given to reduce antibodies, as well as to prepare for thymectomy. Patients may become temporarily weaker after taking *prednisone*, while others may have significant improvement in disease symptoms.

Immunosuppressant drugs, such as *imuran*, may also be used to suppress the activity of the immune system. The effects of these drugs are slow (over a year), and symptoms may recur once the drug is discontinued.

Plasma exchange, which involves an exchange of the plasma (blood) with another healthy individual, is a temporary treatment to increase muscle strength prior to surgery, or to treat temporarily severe symptoms and conditions.

According to Western medicine, steroid medications, such as corticosteroid drugs, are medically necessary to treat many conditions and diseases, including lupus, multiple sclerosis, and *myasthenia graves*. But steroid medications have major effects on the metabolism of calcium and bone, which may lead to severe bone loss, osteoporosis, and bone fractures. As a matter of fact, high dosage of steroid medications can cause rapid bone loss, up to as much as 15 percent per year. If you are on steroids, you are more than twice as likely to have a fracture on the spine or the ribs as compared to a person not taking steroids. In addition, there are even different rates of bone loss among individuals on corticosteroids. Bone loss occurs most rapidly in the first six months after starting oral steroid medications. After 12 months of chronic steroid use, there is a slower rate of bone loss. Fracture risk generally increases as the daily doses of steroid medications increase, although not all patients who take steroid medications experience bone loss.

Other adverse side effects of steroid medications are

elevation of blood pressure, weight gain, decreased resistance to infection, indigestion, thinning of skin, and potential development of cataracts and glaucoma.

Four factors should be carefully considered prior to the use of steroids, especially if your *myasthenia gravis* is related only to ocular muscles:

- Can steroids improve or eradicate your autoimmune disease symptoms?

- Are there other safer forms of therapy to treat your *myasthenia gravis*?

- Does the severity of the symptoms warrant the risk of steroid adverse effects?

- Do steroids reduce the chance of a relapse of your autoimmune disease?

It stands to reason that the high risk of taking pharmaceutical drugs to treat only the symptoms without producing a lasting cure may not warrant the continuation of the medications over a long period.

Therefore, have second thoughts about continuing your medications indefinitely. Instead, believe in the miracle of self-healing

As previously mentioned, **Albert Einstein** once said: "There are two ways to live: you can live as if nothing is a miracle; you can live as if everything is a miracle." Believing that you can cure your *myasthenia gravis* is living your life as if everything is a miracle. Yes, self-healing of *myasthenia gravis* is a miracle of life. Even Western doctors are taught in medical schools that illnesses are self-limiting—that is to say, we can get better on our own. If that is the case, then self-healing is not a myth, but a reality—and a miracle at that.

Therefore, no cure for autoimmune diseases is only a myth, and not a reality. However, the cure does not come from pharmaceutical drugs.

The bottom line: Set your goal to *ultimately* stop all medications. It may take weeks, months, or even years, but that should be your *ultimate* goal in your health pursuit to overcome your autoimmune disease.

Do not stop all your medications right away; that is not safe.

Talk to your doctor first about all your concerns. Express your wish to reduce your medications slowly and gradually.

If your doctor does not agree to your suggestion, look for another naturopathic doctor. Seek second or even third opinion if necessary.

No matter what, make it your ultimate objective to stop *all* medications *eventually*.

The Dangers of Drugs

Millions of people are suffering needlessly as a direct consequence of the unconscionable zeal of the pharmaceutical industry to rake up billions of dollars of profit aided and abetted by scientists and researchers who have been paid handsomely, even to the extent of falsifying tests and research results in some cases.

Not too long ago, three of the top executives of Purdue Pharma pleaded guilty to criminal charges of misleading the public on the risk of addiction and abuse associated with the painkiller drug *OxyContin*. That was only another of the many scandals of pharmaceutical companies doctoring research findings of the safety of drugs and masking their undesirable side effects.

For decades, unreliable drug tests have abounded in the medical and pharmaceutical research community, not only in the United States but also in other parts of the world.

It is not uncommon for pharmaceutical companies to "influence" researchers through coercion, incentive, and even threat, to produce the desired results in clinical trials. Fabricating data, such as in the case of *OxyContin*, is no surprise to the pharmaceutical industry.

Clinical trials, usually involving a small number of people, may not truly reflect the outcome of those who will ultimately be using those drugs after their approval by FDA.

In addition, drugs tested on some animal models may be biased and even irrelevant on humans. An artificially induced disease in non-human animal models may yield results incompatible to a spontaneous, naturally occurring human disease. In short, there is no absolute safety or reliability of many pharmaceutical drugs that are readily available to the public.

The pharmaceutical companies and the FDA have convinced not only the medical establishment but also the gullible public that costly drugs are the only answers to all their health problems, despite their dubious track records and often-deadly side effects.

The use, misuse, and abuse of drugs account for 250,000 to 500,000 deaths each year in the United States. And do you still believe that pharmaceutical drugs provide *all* the possible answers to your health problems? **Dr. O. W. Holmes**, Professor of Medicine, Harvard University, had this to say regarding pharmaceuticals putting you in harm's way: "If all the medicine in the world were thrown into the sea, it would be bad for the fish and good for humanity." **Dr. Holmes'** statement speaks volumes of the potential harm in using pharmaceuticals.

When you give your body a drug that replaces a substance your body is capable of making itself, your body then becomes weaker, not stronger, and begins not only to manufacture *less* of that substance, but also to become *more* dependent on the outside source, which is usually the drug you have been taking.

Unfortunately, no drug can give you insight into the circumstance that created your problems. At best, it can only temporarily reduce the symptoms or physical pain created by your medical condition. A drug "cures" your symptoms at the expense of creating *more* potential symptoms further down the road. For a while, you may be symptom-free, but soon enough new symptoms may emerge, requiring yet a more potent drug to deal with them, and thus forming a vicious cycle of taking more toxic pharmaceutical drugs.

Remember, there is no miracle cure, only natural self-healing, which is holistic health of the body, the mind, and the soul.

According to **Dr. John Tilden**, author of *TOXEMIA*, the first and only cause of disease is *toxemia*, which is the accumulation of toxic wastes over a long period of time. In other words, toxicity retained and stored in our bodies is the common denominator for the causes of all human diseases, including autoimmune diseases.

The Controversy of Flu Shots

In addition to the dangers of drugs in treating autoimmune diseases, including *myasthenia gravis*, there is controversy regarding flu shots. Should you or should you not get a flu shot?

Why does a government health agency try so hard every

year to convince you to get a flu shot? Is it really out of concern for your health? You just wonder. The fact is that the government purchases and distributes most flu vaccines, and very often *overstocks* them. Understandably, the government will always be promoting extensively and enthusiastically the benefits of a flu shot. The government does not want you to go drug free, no more than the pharmaceutical companies behind.

Seniors, in particular, are often recommended to take flu shots. But are they really safe and effective?

In a February 2005 issue of the *Archives of Internal Medicine*, researchers for the National Institute of Allergy and Infectious Diseases compared flu-related mortality among older people to rates of immunization. Their findings were quite surprising: during the past quarter century, immunization rates for the elderly had climbed substantially, while the elderly flu-related mortality rate had stayed the same. In other words, the authorities had *overstated* the benefits of a flu shot among the elderly population.

The truth of the matter is that there is no guarantee that the flu viruses selected for the vaccine will be the identical strains circulating during a given flu season. In fact, there have been many instances of the vaccine not having included some of the strains of the flu currently reported by doctors in the medical community. Moreover, the flu virus may not directly cause the majority of illnesses characterized by fever, fatigue, cough, and aching muscles. In fact, many non-flu viruses may have similar flu-like symptoms.

Vaccines contain killed or less-virulent viruses, bacteria and chemical extracts to stimulate your immune reaction against these organisms. Because more and more reports have cited instances of vaccine failure, manufacturers have made their vaccines *more potent*, which means adding more toxic chemicals. Their long-term adverse side effects may far outweigh their immediate benefits.

The problem with this preventive approach is that in the very young, the nutritionally deficient, and the elderly, *over-stimulating* the immune system may have an opposite effect: it can *paralyze* the immune system.

In addition, the brain may also become over-stimulated into producing free radicals in an effort to kill these make-believe invading organisms.

Who are being targeted? The flu vaccine is generally recommended for persons aged 65 and older, as well as those with a weak immune system and those with medical conditions who could otherwise experience more serious complications from the flu.

Medical journals have reported broad differences in the effectiveness of flu shots for the elderly, ranging from zero to 85 percent. The Center for Disease Control (CDC) stated that 90 percent of deaths from flu occurred among the elderly. Considering that nearly 65 percent of all deaths (from any cause) normally occur in that age group, it is nearly impossible to prove that flu shots significantly increase the life expectancy in that group. The fact is that most people, whether young or old, will mostly recover from the flu without hospitalization or complications. A serious concern of flu shots among the elderly is the increased risk for Alzheimer's disease, according to some research studies.

The final word of wisdom is to avoid using pharmaceutical drugs, which are dangerous chemicals. Do not readily reach out for over-the-counter drugs for your everyday ailments and disorders. Make your own decision whether you should have a flu shot or not now that you are already afflicted with an autoimmune disease that weakens your immune system. The choice is all yours! After all, it is your health, and the symptoms of *myasthenia gravis* are what you may have to confront for the rest of your life.

FIVE

INTERNAL CLEANSING

A Toxic Body

Myasthenia gravis is a disease or disorder caused by the malfunctioning of the immune system. It is partially a result of the accumulated toxins in the body, impairing and weakening the entire immune system.

It is an indisputable fact that pharmaceutical drugs are toxic chemicals. Although they may be effective in temporarily removing some of the undesirable symptoms of a disease, they also have long-term adverse side effects. Therefore, carefully consider the trade-off. The ultimate goal is always to eliminate the use of *all* pharmaceutical drugs.

Sources of Toxins

All these years, knowingly or unknowingly, you may have poisoned your own body with toxins coming from many different sources: industrial wastes; pesticides and herbicides from agricultural products; exhaust fumes from factories and automobiles; food contamination; toxic pharmaceuticals; polluted waters; irradiation from excess use of cell phones, microwave ovens, power plants, radio and satellite transmissions; chemicals in food processing; toxic emotions and negative thoughts. Your body may have ingested these toxins through *absorption*, *consumption*, *inhalation*, and *radiation*, creating health hazards to your immune system. All these toxins have accumulated and remained in your body.

Heavy metals, such as aluminum, cadmium, lead, and mercury, can also cause damages to your immune system. Minerals, which make up approximately four percent of your total body weight, are essential for your immune system and energy production. However, heavy metals can also damage your DNA, adversely change the neurons in your brain, elevate your cholesterol level and blood pressure, as well as deplete your bones of calcium and other minerals. They all play a pivotal role in damaging your immune system, leading to the development of your autoimmune disease.

Common Symptoms of a Toxic Body

The toxins in your body may manifest themselves physically, mentally, and spiritually in the form of bad breath, chronic constipation, chronic fatigue, frequent gas and bloating, hemorrhoids, irritability, mental and spiritual lethargy, overweight, depression, and recurrent headaches or migraines.

These symptoms should not be taken lightly: they often indicate imbalance in the body that may affect your immune system, and thus further aggravating your *myasthenia gravis* symptoms.

Internal Cleansing

Internal cleansing is detoxification, which involves *dislodging* your body toxins and waste products from within and between cells and joints, and then *transporting* these wastes from your body for removal.

Different Ways of Detoxification

There are different ways by which your body can get rid of its toxins:

Fasting to detoxify

Fasting is internal cleansing and rejuvenation—one of the most effective and efficient ways to detoxify your body of its toxins. Fasting is to recovery, as sleep is to recuperation.

Fasting is *voluntary* abstinence from food and drink, except water, for an extended period. Fasting is the *best* way to detoxify your body.

<u>The benefits of fasting</u>

Fasting has many benefits, especially for the immune system.

Fasting activates the immune system in your body to protect you from disease, especially preventing the development of an autoimmune disease.

Fasting accelerates the *self-healing* process of your body because fasting temporarily stops the continuing work of your digestive system, and therefore instrumental in reserving that energy for your internal self-healing process.

By conserving the energy otherwise used in digesting food, fasting provides you with *more*, and not less, energy, contrary to the myth that fasting makes your body weak. Remember, eating and digesting food expends your energy too.

Fasting relieves the burden of not only your digestive tract, but also your liver and kidneys, which have to work extra hard to remove additives and toxins accumulated in your body through improper eating. Fasting removes the underlying cause of any *chronic disease* you may have by removing the toxins, not just the symptoms, as in the case of medications.

Fasting may alleviate your *body pain* and rid your body of any drug dependence. Fasting facilitates you, if you are a smoker, to quit smoking during a fast. Nicotine damages the immune system.

The process of fasting

Eat more vegetables and fruits prior to a fast. Reduce the consumption of meat, and refrain from eating any meat the day before a fast.

On the *first* day, you may feel pangs of hunger, with a white coating on your tongue. This is just a natural response of the body to the cessation of eating. On the first day, you may experience physical weakness, hunger, and food craving. The first day of a fast is most challenging and difficult to endure.

On the *second* day, you may begin to feel gradual dissipation of hunger, with more white coating on your tongue. The discomfort is less severe than the first day of your fast

On the *third* day you may or may not feel *complete* disappearance of hunger and the clearance of coating on your tongue.

The first three days of a fast are most challenging. However, once the challenge is overcome, you are well on the way to rejuvenation of your entire body. From my own experience, after the first three days, you do NOT feel any hunger, and that is the truth. The only hurdle you need to overcome is the first three days of your fast. Remember, **Jesus**, too, fasted for forty days.

What to do during a fast

- Drinking plenty of water is required since your body may easily become dehydrated due to the discharge of body fluids.

- Continue your normal daily routine activities, but avoid all strenuous activities, especially those outdoor ones. Exercise as normal.

- Bathe more frequently. Brush your body to stimulate your skin to rid toxins from your body.

- Stop taking your daily vitamin supplements while you are fasting.

- Consult your doctor to see if you may stop some of the medications you are currently taking.

- Stop smoking if you are a smoker. Now is as good a time as any to quit smoking for good, given that nicotine is most damaging to your immune system, and thus affecting your *myasthenia gravis* symptoms.

How to break a fast

Break a fast on fruits and vegetables juice. Eating an apple is ideal for breaking a fast.

Continue to drink plenty of water after a fast.

Gradually increase your intake of solid food. Eat slowly and chew thoroughly. Overeating too soon may cause abdominal pain and even vomiting.

Avoid taking salt and pepper immediately after a fast, lest they damage your stomach lining.

Remember, the longer the fast, the less you should eat at the *first* meal.

Duration of a fast

A *clear* tongue and *clean* breath are good indications that the cleansing is more or less complete.

The length of a fast depends very much on an individual. The following is just a general guideline for you to follow:

- A one-day fast, as often as required, preferably weekly, for good health maintenance

- A three-to-four-day fast for general health and well being, several times a year

- A two-week fast for complete internal cleansing, every year or so

- A three-week fast (or even longer) for curing a specific disease, under the supervision of a physician.

It is suggested that you begin with a short fast first, and then proceed to a longer fast for complete internal cleansing of your whole body.

Breathing to detoxify

Breathing is the only body function that you can perform both consciously and unconsciously.

The way you breathe is connected to your body and mind. For example, when you are anxious or angry, your breathing becomes quick and shallow—that reduces your body's natural capability to detoxify.

You can *consciously* change your breathing patterns to relax your body and mind to enhance detoxification. Use your *diaphragmatic breathing* (see **page 115**). By holding in your abdominal muscles while pushing out your lower rib cage to expand your diaphragm in your inhalation, you not only acquire *complete breath* (that is, inhaling more oxygen) but also achieve internal cleansing by pumping more lymphatic fluid throughout the body and circulatory systems.

Skin brushing to detoxify

Skin brushing, an external way to detoxify the body, is an effective time-honored method to increase blood and lymphatic circulation to remove dead skin cells, and rid your body of toxins, especially through its pores.

Brush your entire body daily with a natural-bristle dry-skin brush. Be persistent, and the initial discomfort will dissipate after a while when your body has become accustomed to the abrasive effects of brushing.

Foot patches to detoxify

The use of foot patches is an easy and unobtrusive way to assist your body in the removal of a myriad of pollutants that invade your body on a daily basis, as well as the health-repressive toxins that prevent your body from achieving the true wellness you really should be experiencing.

According to Chinese medical knowledge, the human body has over 360 acupuncture points, with more than 60 of them found on the *soles* of the feet alone. Your feet, also known as the "second heart," contain the reflective zones of your internal organs, where your body toxins accumulate and dissipate.

For centuries, Chinese medical studies have held the view that due to gravity, toxins tend to go downwards in your body during the day, accumulating from the tips of the toes to the ankles.

Accordingly, when applied to the soles of your feet *overnight*, these foot patches not only warm up to open pores of the skin but also stimulate the reflex zones on your soles to draw out and absorb accumulated wastes from the blood and lymph systems in your body under osmotic pressure.

When lying horizontally, your body fluids collect in your head and feet. There is an acupuncture point on each of the sole of your feet, known as "gushing water spring," through which excess toxins and moisture from your body will be excreted into the foot patches. By applying foot patches on your feet while sleeping, you may be able to extract toxins from your body through the process of osmosis in the form of moisture onto your soles, and then into the foot patches.

Foot patches are obtainable on the Internet or in Chinese drug stores. Get them to remove toxins from your body.

Hydrotherapy to detoxify

Water is an invaluable nutrient to every living thing on earth. Every cell of your body requires water to carry nutrients and energy to it, as well as to transport toxins and waste products from it.

Always drink enough water. Drink a cup of water as soon as you get up in the morning, not your tea or coffee as your first drink.

According to a survey, only 30 percent of Americans drink at least eight eight-ounce glasses of water a day. Make sure you drink *enough* water, which is more than eight eight-ounce glasses a day. One of the main reasons why people do not drink enough water is that they don't enjoy the taste of plain water; another reason is that they don't have time, especially if they don't feel thirsty (when they *feel* thirsty, they are already dehydrated without knowing it).

According to the Human Nutrition Center at Rockefeller University, water is the best choice for proper hydration.

Drink water on schedule, such as every two hours or so, even if you don't feel thirsty.

Avoid all fruit juices (pasteurized and processed), carbonated beverages (high in phosphoric acid—bone loss; all artificial sweeteners and additives—compromised immunity), and all dehydrating beverages (coffee, tea, carbonated soda with caffeine, beer, wine and other alcoholic drinks).

The bottom line: Drink more water to flush out toxins for internal cleansing.

Unclean water is damaging to health. Always drink only pure water in order to reduce the load on your liver.

When you drink commercial water with additives, carbonation, flavorings, sweeteners, your liver must also work *overtime* to filter them before the water can be absorbed by your body to carry out its proper functions, one of which is to flush out the toxins and wastes from your body system.

The circulating system of blood and lymphatic fluids is vital to all your organs, tissues, and cells in that it enables the removal of waste products from your body.

Hydrotherapy involves alternating application of hot and cold water aimed at increasing your blood flow to different tissues of your body. Take a very hot shower immediately followed by a very cold one, and repeat the process two or three times a day. After the hydrotherapy, snuggle into your bed, staying warm for half an hour or so. With hydrotherapy, you will feel completely refreshed and rejuvenated.

Hydrotherapy provides detoxification benefits to your entire circulating system:

- The alternating hot and cold water opens up pores in your skin for more effective elimination.

- Blood flow increases circulation to your intestines in the abdomen (an empty stomach yielding the best result), thereby promoting digestion.

- The filtering organs of your chest and abdomen are relaxed through the induced circulation.

- The nerves along your spinal cord also become stimulated and relaxed.

Exercise to detoxify

Exercise not only stimulates blood circulation and the

movement of lymphatic fluids, but also promotes the reduction of fat reserves, thereby instrumental in facilitating the removal of toxins stored in your body.

Low-impact aerobic exercise, such as jumping rope or on a bouncer, can significantly improve your body's circulation to enhance detoxification.

Understandably, your weak muscles may make it difficult for you to exercise. Do simple yoga, tai-chi, or qi-gong exercise not only to promote flexibility of muscles but also to increase muscular strength.

Foods to detoxify

Use foods for regular body detoxification, further rejuvenation, and daily maintenance. Some of the top detox foods to help your immune system are as follows:

Apple

An apple a day keeps the doctor away. There is much truth in that: apple is a powerful antioxidant and toxin remover due to its vitamin C and its fiber and pectin. Eat an apple everyday to keep your immune system healthy and strong.

Alfalfa sprouts

Alfalfa sprouts are excellent "health food." Recent research shows that in addition to being a superb source of nutrients, they also have important *cleansing* ability due to their concentrated amounts of phytochemical (plant compounds).

You can grow your own alfalfa sprouts at your home. Just buy some organic alfalfa seeds, put them in a jar, wash and rinse them two or three times a day, and you will have your fresh sprouts in a few days. Sprout some alfalfa seeds at home for your daily salad or soup.

Fresh alfalfa sprouts are also obtainable at some supermarkets.

Artichoke

Artichoke increases your bile production to facilitate your bowel movement. Steam artichoke and serve with a little melted butter.

Avocado

Avocado is rich in glutathione antioxidant, which is effective in removing toxins due to too much alcohol consumption. Eat an avocado for breakfast; it is filling and saves you time.

Beets

Beets help you detoxify your *liver* and *blood* while providing important support nutrients to your body. By providing nutrients critical to liver function and healthy kidneys, beets break down toxins before they accumulate in your liver. In addition, the vitamins and other nutrients contained in beets also enable proper fat absorption, transportation, and metabolism. Include fresh beets in your vegetable juice or salad.

Burdock

Burdock, a carrot-like root grown in China, Europe, and the United States, has a sweet taste and a sticky texture. It is a good source of minerals and essential oils. As such, burdock serves as a staple vegetable in Japan.

Burdock, with its potent anti-bacterial and anti-fungal properties, is a popular folk medicine around the world. As a main source for a variety of herbal preparations, it serves also as a diuretic and, more recently, as a tea to fight cancer (*Essiac* tea in the treatment of cancer and a number of other maladies).

Burdock is a potent "blood purifier" which clears toxins from your bloodstream by enhancing the function of many organs of elimination, including your liver, kidneys and bowels. For example, it induces sweating as an aid in neutralizing and eliminating toxins, thereby instrumental in helping your kidneys filter uric acid from your bloodstream.

Put fresh burdock in your soup, or make a drink of burdock by simmering it in boiling water for 10 minutes (you can repeat the process until its taste is gone). Daily consumption of burdock is highly recommended for your daily internal cleansing.

Green barley

The young barley leaf is a green cereal grass that contains the greatest and most perfectly balanced concentration of nutrients found in nature: enzymes, minerals, many vitamins, including vitamin C, vitamin A, and B vitamins, amino acids, essential fatty acids, carotenoids, bioflavonoids and chlorophyll. The chlorophyll in green barley has the ability to break down carbon dioxide and release oxygen, thereby enabling the destruction of anaerobic bacteria.

Green barley, in addition to its natural form, is available in capsules or powder.

Cruciferous vegetables

Brussels sprouts, cabbage, cauliflower, and spinach are all effective in enhancing your liver in its production of enzymes for your digestion and elimination. Eat them as much and as often as you can, either cooked or raw.

Garlic

Garlic contains allicin, which is a potent purifier of mercury and other toxic chemicals found in most food additives. In addition, garlic alkalizes the body, making it more efficient in resisting disease. Put crushed garlic in all your cooking. If you wish to remove the odor from the unpleasant breath due to garlic, chew some fresh parsley for a fresher breath.

Kiwi fruit

Like avocado, kiwi fruit is loaded with glutathione. In addition, it is rich in vitamin C. It is also a powerful antioxidant to protect your immune system.

Seaweed

Seaweed contains high doses of minerals, such as calcium, iodine, iron, and magnesium, which bind with radioactive wastes from polluted soils and waters, according to research at McGill University in Canada. Seaweed is an inexpensive sea vegetable. Use seaweed in your daily soup.

Watercress

Watercress increases detox enzymes in your body. It is especially effective in removing carcinogens from smokers, according to a United Kingdom research study. Steam or put watercress in your soup.

Herbs to detoxify

Your body is a self-cleaning mechanism, which utilizes your liver, kidneys, urine, feces, breath, and sweat to detoxify your toxins.

Herbs can provide you with safe, natural, and time-tested ways to improve the natural functions of your body through their natural cleansing processes.

Some of the most common herbs for detoxification include: black walnut, cascara sagrada, cayenne, dandelion, echinacea, fennel seed, Indian rhubarb root, licorice root, milk thistle, psyllium husk, red clover, slipper elm inner bark, and yarrow. All these herbs can be obtained on the Internet.

Holistic detoxification

For detoxification to be effective, a holistic approach is required. The body, the mind, and the spirit of an individual are all inter-connected. For this reason, holistic detoxification is the only way to optimum self-cleansing for a healthy immune system.

The spirit also plays an important role. Fasting, for example, is more than a matter of willpower: it involves a deepening of faith and the capability to let go. Fasting is a spiritual act of the mind to detoxify the body. The spirit affects how you react to anxiety, anger, frustration, and other everyday negative emotions that may adversely increase the toxicity in your body because your toxic thoughts are stored in your subconscious mind, which in turn controls your conscious mind. You are what you think: you become your toxic thoughts. Therefore, the role of the spirit in holistic detoxification cannot be overstressed.

SIX

FOODS AS MEDICINE

Free radicals, in the form of radiation stress, chemical stress, and emotional stress, damage your body cells. Always reduce free radicals through detoxification.

Given the optimum environment, your body cells can replicate themselves throughout your lifespan because they are most resilient and rejuvenating.

If you have reduced or stopped your medications, and you have also been detoxifying your body, now is the time to use foods as medicine for recovery and rejuvenation to further promote the self-healing process.

Foods for Acid-Alkaline Balance

Your body cells need an optimum environment for replication and rejuvenation. They need a balanced acid-and-alkaline environment.

Acid and alkaline are substances that have opposing qualities. Your body functions at its best when the pH is optimum, which is slightly alkaline. The pH of your blood, tissues, and body fluids directly affects the state of your cellular health, and hence your immune system.

The pH scale ranges between one and fourteen. *Seven* is considered neutral. Anything *below* seven is considered *acidic*, while anything *above* seven is considered *alkaline*. Deviations above or below a 7.30 and 7.40 pH range can signal potentially serious and even dangerous symptoms, forewarning you of a disease in process.

When your body is too acidic, the tissues of your cells are forced to relinquish their alkaline reserves, depleting them of alkaline minerals, which are the components of the tissues themselves.

The acute shortage of alkaline minerals will lead to disease and the malfunctioning of the immune system, causing an autoimmune disease.

Acidification

Acidification may come from:

- Excess intake of foods containing great amounts of acid

- Insufficient elimination of acid by the body through the kidneys (urination) and the skin (sweating)

Not too much acid can actually stay in the bloodstream, and, accordingly, any excess is directed to other body organs and tissues, where it can accumulate. Too much acidification makes your body sick:

Acid corrosion

The corrosive nature of acid irritates your body organs, causing inflammation (which is often a source of body pain), pain, and hardening of tissues.

Acidic sweat may cause skin allergy, especially in areas where sweat seems to accumulate, such as the armpits.

Acidic urine may also cause infection and inflammation in the urinary tract, resulting in bladder problems.

Acidification not only causes lesions of the mucous membranes (e.g. your respiratory system), making them vulnerable to infections, but also impairs the immune system.

Decreased enzyme activity

Acidification decreases the activity of enzymes in the body, which are responsible for proper digestion of foods and assimilation of nutrients.

Loss of minerals

Loss of minerals may result in the following: bone loss (osteoporosis); brittle bones (hip fracture); joint inflammation (arthritis); hair loss (baldness); split fingernails; dry skin and wrinkles.

Sources of Acidification

Contemporary lifestyle is the main cause of excess acidification in body cells, which may ultimately lead to diseases.

Diet

Diet is the main contributor to excess acidification in the body. The main sources of acid from foods are: cereals (good for the food industry, not for the health); sugars (bad for the body's metabolism); animal proteins (difficult for complete digestion and assimilation by the body).

The main sources of acidification from drinks are: alcohol, coffee, sodas, sugary drinks (often disguised as health drinks), and tea.

Tobacco

Tobacco smoke causes acidification in the respiratory system.

Quit smoking now, if you are still a smoker!

Exercise

Too much exercise (more may not necessarily be better), or the lack of it, may lead to acidification.

Stress

Stress in everyday life and living may cause physiological disturbances, resulting in acidification of your body system.

Diseases Caused by Acidification

Diseases caused by too much acidification are related to the following:

- The immune system

- The skin—allergies and rashes

- The respiratory system—bronchitis, colds, flu, laryngitis

- The nervous system—chronic fatigue, mental depression (due to deficiency in alkaline minerals, including calcium, magnesium, and potassium)

- The urinary system (due to lesions in mucous membranes of the urinary tract).

Acidification is often the inability of the body to metabolize a particular nutrient, such as sugar and animal protein. The wisdom is to avoid sugar totally and reduce the intake of animal protein, both of which are the main culprits of excess acidification in the body.

Foods rich in weak acids, such as fruits, vinegar, and yogurt, are normally quite easy to oxidize, contributing to a large number of alkaline elements in the body. However, if you experience poor oxidation in these foods, your metabolism debility may make you prone to acidification. There are certainly no hard-and-fast rules governing how these weak-acid foods may become acidic or alkaline for different individuals.

Get rid of your sugar addiction.

Symptoms of Excess Acidification

Too much acid in your body may result in some of the following symptoms: acid regurgitation; acidic sweat or dry skin; brittle and fungal nails; conjunctivitis; cracks at the corners of the lips; diarrhea; frequent headaches; insomnia; irritability; leg crams and spasms; lack of energy; lower body temperature; pimples; runny nose; and weight loss.

Measuring Acid-Alkaline Levels

Measure the acid-alkaline levels in you body by

performing a simple urine test with litmus paper (obtainable at pharmacies).

Reduce or eliminate acidification in your body by the following:

- Change your lifestyle: make it *less* stressful.

- Adjust your diet for more alkaline foods and drinks.

- Consume medicinal plants to promote the flow of urine (diuretics) and to increase the production of sweat.

- Take daily alkaline mineral supplements to facilitate internal cleansing.

- Go on a regular water or juice fast to enhance elimination of toxins lodged in the deep tissues of your body.

- Exercise moderately to prevent acidification.

Foods to Balance Acid-Alkaline Levels

Your diet is the primary source that determines your acid-alkaline levels in your body.

All the foods you eat can be divided into three main groups:

Acidifying foods

Acidifying foods are characterized by their high protein content, and/or fats, including the following: meat, poultry, fish and seafood; eggs; cheese; vegetable oils; whole grains;

beans, such as broad bean, chickpeas, peanuts, soybeans, and white beans; bread, pasta, and cereals; sweets and sugars, including brown sugar and honey; sugary drinks and sodas; alcohol, coffee, and tea.

Your digestion of protein produces amino acids (containing acid minerals, such as phosphorus and sulfur) during digestion, and uric acids during acidic degradation.

You utilize fat in the form of fatty acids, and your digestion of saturated fat is often incomplete, resulting in toxic acid substances that contribute to acidification.

Your digestion of glucose may be adversely affected by inadequate or poor metabolism, turning originally alkaline elements into acidic ones.

Your consumption of too much sugar strains your body metabolism in converting it into energy, and thus creating more acid in the process.

In summary, consume *less* acidifying food.

Acid foods

Acid foods may be alkalizing if your body's metabolism is efficient. In other words, if your body can easily metabolize and oxidize them, these foods can be transformed into alkaline elements, making your body more alkaline, instead of more acidic.

Acid foods contain a good deal of acid, and are acidic in taste, including the following: blueberries, raspberries, and strawberries; oranges, grapefruit, lemons, Mandarin oranges, and tangerines; sweet fruits, such as watermelon; unripe fruits; acid vegetables, such as rhubarb, tomato, and watercress; honey; vinegar; and yogurt.

Always eat the fruit, instead of drinking its juice. The reason is that alkaline minerals are present in the pulp; the juice without the pulp is only more acidic.

Cooking fruits does not remove their acidity.

Alkalizing foods

Alkalizing foods contain little or no acid substances, and they do not produce acids when metabolized by your body. Alkalizing foods include the following: green vegetables; colored vegetables (except tomato); chestnut; potato; avocado; black olives; bananas; dried fruits; almonds and Brazil nuts; milk; alkaline mineral waters; and cold-pressed oils.

Potato, especially its juice, is good for stomach acidity and ulcers. It is often an ideal alternative to acidifying cereal grains.

Dried fruits are alkalizing because much of the acid is removed through the drying process. Eat more dried fruits.

Alkalizing medicinal plants

Black currant

Black currant fruits are a good source of vitamin C and other vitamins and minerals, including an omega-6 fatty acid to increase blood flow, to decrease blood clotting, and to reduce inflammation (often a source of many types of body pain).

Black currant seed oil is especially good for rheumatoid arthritis, which is an autoimmune disease, due to its anti-inflammatory properties in decreasing the morning stiffness in the joints.

According to the *British Journal of Rheumatology*, black currant oil is effective because of a reduction in the secretion of the inflammatory cytokines (a source of inflammation).

Black currant seed oil is also beneficial to cardiovascular disease due to the presence of its omega-6 fatty acids.

Black currant seed oil helps reduce the severity of menstrual cramps due to the inflammatory omega-6 fatty acids.

According to the Skin Study Center in Philadelphia, black currant seed oil helps with dry skin disorders. The gamma-linoleic acid (GLA) in black currant protects against water loss that contributes to itching and other symptoms associated with dry skin.

Burdock

Burdock is a plant native to Asia and Europe, which has become available to all parts of the world. Ancient Chinese and Indian herbalists always used burdock to treat respiratory infections, abscesses, and joint pain. The root of burdock is one of the primary sources of most herbal preparations. Eat burdock every day to have a healthy immune system to eliminate many of the symptoms of your *myasthenia gravis*

Cranberry

Cranberry has been in use since the Iron Age, but the Romans were the first to recognize its medicinal values. Cranberry contains anti-asthmatic compounds, and is high in vitamin C and antioxidants.

Scientific studies have shown cranberry to be effective in helping to prevent or eliminate urinary tract infections. This berry is useful in fighting yeast infections, as well as kidney stones and chronic kidney inflammation.

According to a study reported at the 2006 *International*

Association for Dental Research's 84th General Session & Exhibition in Brisbane, Australia, the antioxidant properties of cranberry help fight dental plaque.

Alkalizing energy boosters

Spirulina

Spirulina is a green alga, rich in chlorophyll, containing the highest protein and beta-carotene levels of all green super foods. It is the highest known vegetable source of B-12, minerals, trace elements, cell salts, amino acids, DNA and RNA, and enzymes.

Spirulina helps with digestion, elimination, detoxification, internal cleansing, tissue repair, skin problems, healing, and prevention of degenerative disease. It also promotes longevity. Spirulina is effective in any weight-control diet because its high nutritional value helps satisfying the hidden hunger or deficiencies.

Blackstrap molasses

Blackstrap molasses is an excellent source of iron and calcium, copper, magnesium, manganese, and potassium. It can even reverse gray hair due to its copper content.

Make a healthy drink with a tablespoon of organic blackstrap molasses (mixed in some hot water first) and ¾ cup of soymilk. Add ice.

Cod liver oil

Cod liver oil, which comes from fatty fish, such as salmon and sardines, is rich in vitamin A and vitamin D, and essential omega 3 oils. It enhances the absorption of calcium and maintains a constant level of blood calcium. Cod liver oil also improves brain functions and the nervous system.

In 2005, researchers at the *University of California* reported that Vitamin D might lower the risk of developing different types of cancers, cutting in half the chances of getting breast, ovarian, or colon cancer.

Alkaline supplements

Alkaline supplements should contain calcium (Ca), sodium (Na), silica and copper, and other minerals to aid de-acidification of your body. More importantly, they should contain every mineral in similar proportion to that found in the human body.

Remember, the human body functions synergistically: the whole is greater than the sum of its parts. Every mineral has a crucial role to play in the human anatomy.

Supplement your diet with coral calcium to keep all mineral levels up, as well as in their proper balance.

Food Allergies

Besides using foods to boost and enhance immune system health, it is also important to avoid food allergies.

Research has indicated that many autoimmune disease patients also have food allergies. This research finding of higher rates of allergies in general has led some experts to believe that food allergies may also be the triggering of some autoimmune diseases. Many nutritionists also concur that an anti-inflammatory diet not only may avoid getting another autoimmune disease, but also can alleviate some of the symptoms of an already-existing autoimmune disease. (See **Appendix E**)

Gastrointestinal Tract Infection

Make sure your gastrointestinal tract is thriving. Although your autoimmune disease, such as *myasthenia gravis*, is not directly connected to your stomach, your digestive health is inextricably linked to the source of your autoimmunity. In an unhealthy intestine, the lining may become impaired, and thus allowing larger molecules, such as bacteria and undigested foods, to slip through into the bloodstream. This may trigger an immune reaction.

Therefore, it is also important to cleanse your gastrointestinal tract through diet to prevent antigens from getting into your body system that may further increase the production of antibodies to go after the added antigens, and thus worsening your immune-driven disease symptoms.

Basics of Eating for a Healthy Immune System

There are basics of healthy eating; with a little discipline, they are simple to follow, and may go a long way to improving your immune system.

Eating to Live, Not Living to Eat

You become your food, and your food becomes you, because you are what you eat. What you eat and drink becomes your body chemistry.

Eating Less, Not More

Follow the "three-quarters" rule of eating: stop eating when you are three-quarters full. Never overeat.

Eating Frequently, Not Three Times a Day

You need not follow the habit of eating three times a day. Eat only when you are hungry, not because it is time to eat. Eating smaller meals more frequently is less taxing on your digestive and metabolic systems.

Eating Living Foods, Not Dead Foods

Eat only living foods: fresh, whole, and, preferably, organic foods.

Do not eat processed foods (supermarket foods), which are loaded with colorings, preservatives, and taste enhancers.

Do not eat empty-calorie foods, such as white flour and white sugar: foods are supposed to give you energy and nutrients, not just empty calories.

Also, stop eating foods that damage your thyroid, which is critical to your immune health. Avoid foods that contain goitrogens, which are substances occurring naturally in certain foods that may cause your thyroid gland (goiter) to enlarge. Goitrogens are naturally found in soy, millet, coffee, and cruciferous vegetables, such as broccoli, cauliflower, cabbage, and kale (do not over-consume them; steam them instead of eating them raw). To enhance your thyroid health, take iodized salt (but not too much) and coconut oil. Also, drink plenty of water.

Eating Sea Salt, Not Table Salt

Eat sea salt, which is loaded with minerals. Avoid table salt. Research has shown that increased salt intake proportionately increases cancer risk in the bladder, esophagus, and stomach.

Eating No Refined Sugar

Get your sugar from fruits and vegetables. Stay away from refined sugar.

Artificial sugars, such as aspartame, saccharin, or sucralose, are more dangerous than refined sugar, because they are loaded with chemicals that impair the immune system. Stop your sugar craving and addiction!

Eating Raw Occasionally

For optimum digestion, your body needs enzymes, which are destroyed by heat in cooking. You need not be a vegetarian to go on raw, but vegetarians generally have a better and healthier immune system. An occasional raw duet increases enzyme activities for better digestion and assimilation to enhance your immune system.

Chewing Thoroughly

Chew your food thoroughly—at least 20 times before swallowing. The benefits of thorough chewing are:

- Activating enzymes for better digestion

- Facilitating the absorption of vitamins and nutrients

- Feeling fuller, therefore eating less (better weight control)

- Reducing the production of stomach acid (cause of heartburn).

Smart Cooking

Steaming is the best way to cook. Steam your food to preserve its nutrients. The next best cooking method is stir-fry. Boiling destroys half of the vitamins in vegetables. Deep-frying not only yields fatty foods but also produces trans fat (the worst kind of fat).

Foods for the Immune System

Chlorella

Chlorella is a green single-cell alga cultivated in fresh water ponds. It is one of the best foods for the immune system.

- It has high concentration of chlorophyll.

- It has high source of protein.

- It is the perfect anti-aging food (more than 20 vitamins and minerals, with the essential eight amino acids) for overall health.

- It detoxifies by removing toxins and metals from the body.

Wheat Grass

Wheat grass is another life-giving food for the immune system.

- It is rich in chlorophyll to provide oxygen for the

brain and body tissues.

- It is loaded with enzymes for optimum digestion.

- It absorbs as many as 92 of the known 102 anti-aging minerals from the soil (if grown in organic soil) to boost your immune system.

Wheat grass juice is particularly a superior detoxification agent compared to carrot juice. It enhances digestion, relieves sore throat, keeps the bowels open, reduces blood pressure, and improves the cholesterol levels. Make your own wheat grass juice, or obtain it from a health food store.

Foods to Boost the Immune System

Apples

An apple a day keeps the doctor away. Eat two to three apples a day to keep you healthier for longer. The pectin in apples may do wonders to your health by decreasing your cholesterol levels, facilitating your bowel movements to keep you internally clean, improving lung functions (according to one study, better lung function with eating at least five apples a week), and preventing colon cancer.

Brown Rice

Brown rice is one of the few pain-safe foods (foods that do not trigger body pain). It is one of the best staple foods for lowering high blood sugar (excellent for diabetics), and anti-aging (over 70 oxidants) vitamin E, glutathione peroxidase, coenzyme Q-10

Do not eat white rice, which is stripped of some of its major nutrients.

Garlic

Eat fresh garlic everyday. To overcome its pungency, chew some fresh parsley (rich in vitamin C). The allicin in garlic has the following medicinal properties: combating cancer, lowering cholesterol, preventing atherosclerosis and coronary blockage, reducing blood clot formation, regulating blood sugar, and stimulating the pituitary to produce hormones.

Sea Vegetables

Sea vegetables have more concentrated nutrients (e.g. calcium, iron, and protein) than land vegetables.
Sea vegetables have immense health benefits for the immune system by detoxifying heavy metals, dissolving cysts and tumors, shrinking goiters, and reducing water retention for weight loss.
Add sea vegetables to your salads and soups.

Sweet Potatoes and Yams

Sweet potatoes and yams are rich in beta-carotene, fiber, protein, vitamin C, and DHEA, which is a precursor hormone (dehydroepiandrosterone).

Drinks to Heal the Immune System

Burdock and Daikon Drink

Burdock root has been used as both food and medicine

in Asia and Europe for thousands of years. Recently, it has been used as a nourishing tonic for cancer, liver disease, and rheumatism. Burdock root is a staple diet of the Japanese, who are among the people with the longest lifespan in the world.

Fresh burdock root is available at many greengrocers, Asian supermarkets, and natural food stores in the United States.

Daikon is Japanese radish. Its phytochemicals have recognized healing and anti-carcinogenic properties:

- It cleanses the blood (the kidneys).

- It promotes energy circulation.

- It increases the metabolic rate (a weight-loss remedy in Asia).

- It treats hangovers.

- It decongests the lungs, clears sore throat, colds, and edema.

The burdock and daikon drink can be taken any time, and as much as you like.

Ingredients

- One burdock root (about 24 inches long)

- One daikon with green tops

- One small carrot with green tops

Preparation

- Cut all ingredients into small pieces.

- Place them in a pot with water double the volume of the ingredients.

- Bring to a boil.

- Pour out the content, and drink it.

- You can repeat the process one more time. This time, after bringing it to a boil, reduce heat, and simmer it for another 20 minutes. Let the ingredients steep in the hot water for another 20 minutes before drinking it.

Four Greens Drink

Bitter melon, a popular Asian vegetable, is well known for blood glucose control. It contains a substance similar to bovine insulin, which has been shown in experimental studies to achieve a positive sugar regulating effect by suppressing the neural response to sweet taste stimuli.

Celery is a good source of insoluble fiber as well as essential nutrients, including vitamin C, calcium, and potassium. In addition, it may reduce blood pressure, and block cancer cells.

Cucumber has been associated with healing properties in relation to diseases of the kidney, urinary bladder, liver and pancreas. In addition, cucumber juice is an excellent skin tonic.

Green pepper is loaded with vitamin C (a potent

antioxidant) and beta-carotene (to prevent cataracts).

Make the nutritious four greens drink by juicing them in approximately equal portions. Drink immediately.

Pine Needles Drink

Pine needle drink is a perfect drink made from evergreen pine needles. Select your pine needles by picking the newest green ones from a pine tree. Wash the pine needles thoroughly. Put them in a cloth bag, and steep it in a pot of boiling water—if you don't use a cloth bag, then strain the needles before drinking. Cover and let it sit for 30 minutes.

Pine needle drink is loaded with vitamin C and other nutrients to offer the following benefits: eyesight; fatigue; heart disease; kidney ailments; sclerosis (inflammatory nerve disorder); and varicose veins.

Foods for Balance and Harmony

The Yin and Yang Diet

For centuries, the Chinese have observed the importance of balance and harmony, manifested in the concept of *yin* and *yang* (represented as the *female* and *male*, respectively, or any two opposing forces in Nature that balance and complement each other, resulting in perfect harmony).

The terms *yin* and *yang* describe the opposite yet complementary energy states in the universe. A balance between the two polarities can help you stay in beneficial energy alignment, which is fundamental to wellness. *Yin* embodies negative electrical charge and contractive energy, while *yang* demonstrates positive electrical charge and expansive energy.

The balance of *yin* and *yang* is reflected in the Five Elements, which form the basis of the *yin* and *yang* diet for a healthy immune system.

The Five Elements

This concept of balance and harmony originates from the Five Elements (wood, fire, earth, metal, and water), which not only are fundamental to the cycles of Nature, but also correspond to the different organs of the human body. In addition, each of these elements also corresponds to a different color.

These Five Elements not only balance but also complement each other to create harmony. To illustrate, water nourishes trees or wood, without which there will be no fire, and without fire, there will be no earth, and without earth, there will be no metal; fire heats metal to produce water through condensation, and without metal, there will be no water. These Five Elements are inter-dependent on one another for existence in the form of a cycle of Nature.

Wood corresponding to green

- Eat green vegetables, from asparagus to dark leafy greens, such as spinach.

- Eat green fruits, such as lime, and melon.

- Eat pumpkin seeds.

- Eat green-colored beans, such as lentils, and mung beans; and grains, such as rye.

Fire corresponding to red

- Eat red vegetables, such as hot red peppers and bell peppers, or beets.

- Eat red fruits, such as red apples, or cherries.

- Eat red nuts, such as pecans.

- Eat red-colored beans, such as red lentils, and red beans; and grains, such as buckwheat.

Earth corresponding to orange and yellow

- Eat orange and yellow vegetables, such as pumpkins, squash, and yams.

- Eat orange and yellow fruits, such as mangoes, oranges, and papaya.

- Eat orange and yellow nuts, such as almonds, and cashews.

- Eat orange and yellow beans, such as chickpeas, and grains, such as corn and millet.

Metal corresponding to white

- Eat white vegetables, such as cauliflower, and daikon radish.

- Eat white fruits, such as bananas, and pears.

- Eat white nuts, such as macadamias, and pine nuts.

- Eat white-colored beans, such as soybeans and white beans; and grains, such as barley and rice.

Water corresponding to black, blue, and purple

- Eat dark-colored vegetables, such as black mushroom, eggplant, and seaweed.

- Eat dark-colored fruits, such as blackberries, blueberries, and raisins.

- Eat dark-colored nuts, such as black sesame, and walnuts.

- Eat dark-colored beans, such as black beans and navy beans; and grains, such as black wild rice.

According to the famous *Yellow Emperor's Classic of Medicine*, health and self-healing are contingent on a balance and harmony of all five elemental energies. Therefore, you are recommended to eat a diet that includes vegetables, fruits, nuts, beans and grains of all the five colors in order to initiate the self-healing process of the immune system to heal your *myasthenia gravis*.

Foods to Avoid to Protect the Immune System

Sugar

A recent U.S. Department of Agriculture (USDA) survey revealed that the average American consumes the equivalent of 160 pounds of sugar a year—that is, something like over 50-heaped teaspoons of sugar per person per day.

Avoid all white sugar, corn syrup, Aspartame and Nutrasweet©. Sugar is one of the common toxic foods that stresses the immune system; it is not a health food by any stretch of imagination because it spells toxicity in many ways:

Too much sugar may suppress your immune system and upset your body's mineral balance, making it more acidic.

Too much sugar consumption may cause blood sugar imbalance and food craving, leading to obesity.

Too much sugar may overburden your pancreas, rendering it incapable of clearing sugar from your blood efficiently. This sugar imbalance may potentially lead to diabetes.

Too much sugar intake may cause anxiety, irritability, nervous tension, and even depression due to depletion of your body's B-complex vitamins and minerals, especially for those women progressing to menopause.

Too much sugar consumption may reduce your absorption of good cholesterol (HDLs), while increasing your bad cholesterol (LDLs).

Eating too much sugar is not healthy eating at all. Look at all food and drink labels before you consume them. Any food item loaded with sugar is bad for your immune system.

Unfortunately, sugar is also *hidden* in almost all commercial processed foods and drinks that are available in supermarkets.

Corn syrup, known as glucose syrup outside the United States, comes from cornstarch, composed mainly of glucose. A series of enzymatic reactions is used to convert the cornstarch to corn syrup to sweeten soft drinks, juices, ice cream, whole wheat bread and many other mass-produced foods.

Corn syrup in its liquid form not only keeps foods moist but also prevents them from quickly spoiling. It is good for food manufacturers, but bad for you. Corn syrup is not for healthy eating.

High fructose corn syrup (HFCS) is a modified form of corn syrup that has an increased level of fructose. HFCS is no more or less harmful than other forms of sugar.

Aspartame was accidentally discovered in 1965 as a sweetener.

The dangers of aspartame poisoning have been a well-guarded secret since the 1980s. The research and history of aspartame have attested to aspartame as being a cause of illness and toxic reactions in the human body. There is conclusive evidence that aspartame is a dangerous chemical food additive, and its use during pregnancy and by children is one of the greatest modern health concerns.

Unfortunately, in 1996, aspartame was finally approved by the FDA. It took decades to get the FDA's approval for a good reason—there was, and there is, too much objection to its much controversial safety to the public health. With the blessing from the United States, now aspartame is extensively used in most processed foods—as many as 5,000 food and drug items, including even some nutritional supplements.

Today, millions of people around the world consume products containing aspartame. Its wide popularity is due to its low caloric value as well as its sugar-like taste. In fact, the calories in most processed foods can be substantially reduced, if not eliminated, by using aspartame in place of sugar.

Suggested sugar replacements for healthy eating for a healthy immune system

If you must have sugar in spite of its deadly potentials, consider the following alternatives for a healthier immune system:

Use apple or other sweet fruit juices for many recipes in cooking and desserts. But avoid juices made from "concentrate," which have little or no nutritional value.

Use barley malt made from sprouted barley, or brown rice syrup in bakery.

Use blackstrap molasses, a by-product of sugar refining process, which contains calcium, iron, and B vitamins, and which has about a quarter of the calories of refined sugar.

Use dried fruit puree made from dried organic apricots, cranberries, dates, figs, and prunes that have not been treated with sulfur.

Use fresh carrot juice as a refreshing sweet drink.

Use maple syrup in cooking or as a sweetener. Maple syrup comes from sap of maple tree. Organic pure 100 percent maple syrup is a little expensive but highly recommended.

Use raisins as a sweetener with oatmeal and fruit salad.

Use stewed fruits as desserts.

Use sweet brown rice with raisins as a sweet-tasting meal or dessert.

Use vanilla rice milk to replace milk and sugar in teas and cereals

There are indeed many ways to avoid sugar in your cooking and diet. Wherever possible, avoid sugar.

Dairy Products

Today's milk is no more than a *chemical*, *biological*, and *bacterial* cocktail.

Instead of the old-fashioned fresh green grass feeding

and traditional methods of breeding, modern feeding methods of cows use high-protein, soy-based feeds, and high-technology breeding to produce cows with abnormally large pituitary glands so that they can *artificially* produce much more milk. Just think about *that!*

Today, an average cow may produce 30,000 to 40,000 pounds of milk per year, as opposed to the 2,000 pounds produced by its counterpart half a century ago. Such discrepancy may be due to drugs, antibiotics, hormones, forced feeding plans, and specialized breeding. In 1990, the U.S. Food and Drug Administration approved a genetically engineered hormone injected into dairy cows to make them produce more milk. However, the Canadian government and scientists challenged the safety of that hormone to humans.

Cow's milk is no longer *pure* as it was before. Just think about *what* is in your milk.

Dairy products may play a major role in the development of allergies, asthma, insomnia, and migraine headaches. At least 50 percent of all children in the United States are allergic to cow's milk, and many remain undiagnosed. Dairy products are the leading cause of food allergy, manifested in diarrhea, constipation, and chronic fatigue, although they may not be one of the causes of autoimmune diseases.

Milk also contains powerful *growth hormones*, which may play a major role in human breast cancer. Milk is a hormonal delivery system. If you believe that breast-feeding mothers deliver substances to their infants, then you should understand that milk is a hormonal delivery system, too.

Today, milk is *homogenized*, which means the fat molecules in milk are evenly distributed within the liquid milk such that there is no visible cream separation in the milk. By *artificially* changing nature's natural mechanism, milk proteins are not broken down, and are directly absorbed into your bloodstream without your adequate digestion. Undigested proteins may account for increased rates of cancers, especially breast cancers, and heart disease. This may explain why there is such low incidence of breast cancer in rural China, where there is low consumption of dairy products.

To make matters worse, *synthetic* vitamin D is often fortified and added to homogenized milk to replace the natural vitamin D complex displaced during the process of homogenization.

Synthetic vitamin D is toxic to your liver. Do not believe that your milk "fortified" with vitamin D is a better health food. No, it is not! Some good stuff has been taken out of your milk and is replaced by something not as good. For this reason, milk may not be a health food for healthy eating for everyone.

Normal milk may be bad enough as it is. On top of that, if milk is *pasteurized* (heated to kill bacteria in milk), it is being changed into something other than milk. When milk is pasteurized, much of its enzymes are destroyed in the process, making milk protein even more difficult to digest.

To protect your immune system, stay away from dairy products as much as possible.

Soy

The soybean known today is not the *same* plant traditionally grown in China. Prior to its introduction into the United States, this 20th century version of soybean was *genetically manipulated* in Europe in the 1950s to increase its yield for industrial purposes. In fact, soybean was listed in the 1913 U.S. Department of Agriculture (USDA) handbook not as a food but as an industrial product.

Soy may not be the health food for healthy eating that the food industry claims for the following reasons:

Soy has high concentrations of certain chemicals that combine with essential minerals to deposit insoluble salts difficult for your kidneys to eliminate.

Soy may also adversely affect enzymes and hormones production in your body.

Soy protein is difficult for your digestion. Soybean is a seed. Like all other seeds, soybean is rich in *enzyme inhibitors* (anti-digestive) to protect it from the environment.

Soybean did not serve as a food until about 3,000 years ago when the ancient Chinese introduced the art of *fermentation*, neutralizing enzyme inhibitors and predigesting soybean with several fungus enzymes.

The Chinese did not eat unfermented soybean as they did other legumes, such as lentils, because soybean contains large quantities of natural toxins.

Only after the Chinese mastered the principle of pre-digesting soybean with natural substances to enhance its nutritional value during the Chou Dynasty (1134-246 B.C.) was soybean designated as one of the five sacred grains along with barley, wheat, millet, and rice for healthy eating.

Unfortunately, advances in technology, with the use of harmful chemicals, such as emulsifiers, flavorings, preservatives, and synthetic nutrients, have turned soybean into multiple soy products, while for centuries the Chinese have been consuming soy and its products only as a *small* portion of their healthy eating diet.

The bottom line: Consume soy products, such as soymilk and tofu, only moderately, if you *must*. Remember, soy products are no longer good for the immune system, especially your *myasthenia gravis*.

Hippocrates, the father of modern medicine, once said: "Let food be your medicine; and your medicine, your food." Empower your mind with information, and manage your *myasthenia gravis* with your diet and food choice, given that there is no known cure, according to modern medicine.

SEVEN

LIFESTYLE CHANGES TO HEAL

Cigarette Smoking

Cigarette smoke is a health-wrecker, especially to the immune system. The tar in cigarette smoke is composed of chemicals, poisons, and corrosives, such as hydrogen cyanide and carbon monoxide, which deprive your heart and other organ tissues of essential oxygen for optimum function, in particular, the immune system. Cigarette smoking is one the major triggers of autoimmune diseases.

The Health Hazards

Cigarette smoke produces free radicals that destroy cells and tissues, and hence the ultimate impairment of the immune system

Smoking leads to premature cell-death in the heart, the lungs, and the nervous system—and the ultimate breakdown of the immune system.

Smoking not only promotes the deposits of fat and cholesterol on the walls of arteries, restricting blood flow to the heart and the brain, but also increases the risk of blood clots and stroke.

Smoking causes lung diseases, such as chronic bronchitis (inflammation of the airways) and emphysema (irreversible breakdown of lung tissues), and lung cancer (90 percent of lung cancers are caused by smoking). Men over 35 who smoke are ten times more likely to die of lung diseases.

Secondhand Smoke

Secondhand smoke is as harmful as inhaled smoke.

According to the Environmental Protection Agency, secondhand smoke accounts for some 4,000 lung-cancer deaths a year. If you smoke, your immune system as well as that of your spouse may be adversely affected.

Quitting the Habit

If smoking has already become a habit or an addiction, quit smoking at all cost to protect your immune system.

Nearly 80 percent of smokers who strive to kick the habit will suffer relapses. Quitting is never easy because it may immediately result in the following symptoms: slowing down of heart rate, elevation of blood pressure, development of ulcers, lack of mental concentration, anxiety and depression, drowsiness, and gastrointestinal disturbances, among others.

Quitting may put you in a catch-22 situation. However, the long-term effects of smoking are disastrous to your immune system. Success in quitting is contingent upon the following:

You must make the personal decision to quit smoking as the first and most important step to cure *myasthenia gravis*. Only *you* can decide to quit.

You must overcome the denial that smoking is a systematic suicide. This initiates your desire to make the decision to quit.

You must persist and persevere in taking repeated actions to quit smoking, despite repeated relapses and failures. Remember, **Sir Winston Churchill** once said: "Never, never, never give up!" You must do the same— never, never, never give up quitting smoking!

You must make a commitment to take the necessary actions, and success will be the follow-through.

Alcohol Drinking

Excessive drinking of alcohol may lead to alcoholism, which has led to auto accidents, divorces, loss of employment, and health deterioration, among other disasters in life. Anyway, alcohol is bad for the immune system.

Alcohol dependence may start with being a social drinker, who drinks a little too much. Then comes the use of alcohol for "self-medication" to overcome loneliness and stress, among other psychological and emotional problems in life.

Development of alcohol dependence often comes in different phases:

- From a heavy social drinker, you begin to develop alcohol tolerance.

- During drinking episodes, you may have memory lapses.

- You begin to have little or no control over your drinking.

- You experience prolonged binges of drunkenness, accompanied by both mental and physical complications.

Behavioral signs of alcohol dependence include personality changes, such as irritability, uncontrolled rage, and selfishness.

Physical symptoms include nausea and vomiting, abdominal pain, tingling and trembling sensations, irregular pulse, confusion and memory loss.

Alcoholics require detoxification to overcome withdrawal symptoms experienced after quitting.

Detoxification has to be followed by long-term therapy treatments:

- Medical treatments to deal with withdrawal symptoms and cravings

- Psychological treatments to deal with behavioral and emotional problems (often in a group setting)

- Social treatments to deal with problems at work and at home

Overcome your alcohol addiction at all cost to help you eliminate the symptoms of an autoimmune disease.

Beer Drinking

If you drink more than two glasses of beer a day, you may gradually develop alcohol tolerance, ending up in drinking more. If you have problems with your immune system, abstain from alcohol!

Stress

Stress is your body's response to increased tension. Stress is normal. You need stress to do the following: accepting challenges; concentrating on doing a difficult task; having sex; and making important decisions.

Indeed, stress can be conducive to health. For example, sex creates stress: it increases your pulse rate and heartbeat, and stimulates your brain cells. Stress can be enjoyable, such as physical challenge in competitive sports.

But too much stress can increase your production of hormone epinephrine (and thus wearing out your hormonal glands) with the following effects: blood sugar elevation to produce more energy; breathing rate acceleration to get more oxygen; muscle tension; pulse rate and blood pressure increase; and sweating to cool down the body.

After the initial stressful stimuli, your body should be able to relax, slow down, and return to a state of equilibrium. However, if this does not happen, you become *distressed.*

Stress is the No. 1 factor not only in the cause of many human diseases, but also in the trigger of many autoimmune disease symptoms.

Stress and anger often go hand in hand. They cause hormone imbalance, which may trigger the development of an autoimmune disease.

Chronic stress, which causes your body to maintain physiological reactions for long periods of time, especially with respect to the release of hormones, can lead to depletion of vital nutrients in your body, particularly DHEA (a hormone critical to aging and the immune system), vitamin C, and the B-complex vitamins.

During stress, your body uses its DHEA supply and

impairs the functioning of your body's hormonal glands. According to scientific research, your DHEA levels decrease with age. Therefore, stress is only adding insult to injury.

Vulnerability to stress increases with age. **Robert Sapolsky**, author of *Zebras Don't Get Ulcers*, says you lose your ability to cope with stress as you age, due to elevated blood pressure, which adversely impacts your hormone secretions, and thus creating a vicious cycle of stress and ill health.

To avoid or to decrease the symptoms of an autoimmune disease, learn to cope with stress and deal with anger.

Understand the Causes of Stress in Your Life

Stress may be caused by many factors, including the following:

Financial problems

Finance is one of the main stress factors in contemporary life due to unemployment, not having enough money to make both ends meet, debt from credit cards or gambling, home foreclosure, and unexpected exorbitant medical bills, among others.

To avoid financial stress, learn how to manage your money.

Health problems

The American Academy of Family Physicians once estimated that two-thirds of all family doctor visits are stress-related.

Health problems can be triggered by alcohol, sugar, and tobacco addiction. Chronic health problems are particularly stressful.

Relationships

Relationships are often a source of emotional and psychological problems, such as breakup in a love relationship, separation and divorce, dealing with teenager problems, and coping with aging parents.

Work environment

According to the American Institute of Stress, up to one million employees absence per day are stress-related.

Work environment creates stress due to feeling of being unproductive, inability to concentrate on work, unrealistic and unreasonable demands from employer or co-workers, racial discrimination, and sexual harassment, among others.

Stressful life events

Both special life events—whether they are positive or negative—can be stressful, such as marriage or a wedding, graduation, a new job, buying a home, and even going on a vacation.

Your experience of stress can be *past*, *current*, and *future*.

Past stress (also known as "residual stress") is stress from the past that you cannot overcome completely despite the passage of time.

Current stress is a current state of arousal caused by an existing situation that requires your immediate attention but that you do not enjoy addressing.

Future stress is "anticipatory stress" or worry about what might happen in the future. Residual stress can lead to future stress, passed on from unpleasant past experience.

Ways to Handle Stress

Basically, there are only three different ways to handle stress:

Avoid stress

Avoiding stress is only a temporary solution: it does not solve the very underlying stress problem. Avoiding stress is what is commonly known as the "fight-or-flight" response.

To deal with this type of stress, you may use your innate defensive mechanism to cope with stress by subconsciously distorting the realty. This is tantamount to self-denial of a stressful situation.

Unfortunately, avoidance of stress only reinforces the feeling of inadequacy and perpetuates the vicious cycle of stress. Avoiding or delaying the problem may only intensify the stress further down the road.

Procrastination is another form of this defensive mechanism. Unfortunately, this, too, is only a temporary measure: it does not eradicate the problem itself.

Manage stress

Manage stress by changing the perceptions of stress. Stress is always in the mind's eye, that is, the perceptions.

Relax

Use relaxation techniques to help the body and the mind to cope with stress. (Go to **EIGHT**)

Stress Management

Stress management is essentially about the perceptions of stress. In other words, it is all in the mind's eye: what is stress to one individual may not be stress to another.

The key to managing stress is achieving the right balance between tension and relaxation.

First and foremost, you must identify the main stressors in your life, that is, the *causes* of your stress, and *why* they stress you, and not others

Then, you adopt practical measures to cope with them.

Perceptions of stress

Stress is nothing more than your own perceptions of it. That is to say, it is an *attitude* or a *personal reaction* to certain events and experiences in life.

William Shakespeare rightly said: "There is nothing either good or bad, but thinking makes it so."

John Milton, the famous English poet, also had this to say: "The mind is its own place, and in itself can make a Heaven of Hell, a Hell of Heaven."

Given that stress is no more than your own perceptions, controlling your own perceptions is effective stress management.

Your perceptions of stress are generally based on the following:

Care and value—the more you care about something, the more stressful it is to you.

Choices and options—the more choices and options open to you, the less stressed you are.

Conscientiousness—the more conscientious you are, the more stressed you may become.

Enjoyment—the more you enjoy doing something, the less stressful it is to you.

Responsibility—the more you are responsible for the stressful situation, the more stressed you become.

You can use your subconscious energies to control your perceptions of stress or just about anything in life.

You can also change your perceptions of stress by learning to use positive affirmations to bring about the change.

Long-term measures to manage stress

Chronic (long-term) stress causes your body to have prolonged physiological reactions, precipitating various health problems. Use your conscious adaptive mechanism to adjust to change and to learn to see your stress in perspective. They have long-term impact on copying with stress.

Self-evaluation

Be honest with yourself: what you can do and cannot do. Never overreach yourself to create the unnecessary anxiety and resultant stress. Also, be honest with others: do not wear a mask. To foster a genuine relationship of honesty and integrity, you need to be honest with others, as well as with yourself.

Support, not withdrawal and isolation

Withdrawal and isolation may be consequences of the

inability to cope with stress. Withdrawal and isolation only aggravate the stressful situation. To avoid this:

Join a social group: you must feel accepted and appreciated by others.

Seek a confidante: someone you can confide your deepest feelings of anxiety, fear, and frustration. The confidante can be your spouse, your counselor, or a very close friend.

Choose a supportive environment: be around people who are supportive and encouraging, and who share your views and values. Studies have shown that having a close, supportive network not only reduces stress but also promotes a healthy immune system.

A good diet and a healthy lifestyle

A good diet prevents disease, which may become a stressor in life.

Caffeine and nicotine are known to stimulate the production of *epinephrine*, which accentuates your body's stress response.

Adequate sleep helps you relax both physically and mentally.

Exercise reduces muscular contraction due to poor posture and tension.

(See Relaxation Techniques in **EIGHT**)

Change of situation or environment

A change of situation or environment may help alleviate the stress, such as changing a job, moving to a new place. However, the change itself may call for major decisions, which may also contribute to new stress.

Self-improvement

Learn new skills to deal with difficult situations. Learn to be assertive.

Learn to express your own opinions and beliefs.

Learn to say yes or no in a calm, relaxed, and reasonable manner without violating the rights of others.

Learn to consider your basic rights without having to give reasons or justifications.

Learn to put your own wishes before those of others.

Learn to take responsibility of your own feelings and behavior.

Time management

Good time management means you have time for yourself to relax and recharge your energies.

Good time management means you balance home, work, and leisure effectively such that you have space for yourself.

Procrastination is not just the thief of time but also the stressor in life. Stop your procrastination today!

Stop driving yourself crazy amidst the hassles of contemporary life. Simply learn how to relax and cope with time stress.

Manage stress the Chinese way

Taoism or Tao (also called The Way) is a way of life, which has been practiced in China for thousands of years.

The wisdom of Tao to manage stress in life is succinctly expressed in *Tao Te Ching* ("Te" means "virtuosity" and "Ching" means "classic"). This ancient Chinese classic was written around the 6th century B.C. by the sage **Lao Tzu** ("Lao" means "Old" and "Tzu" means "Master"). It has become one of the most translated works in world literature due to its popularity and the profound wisdom expressed in the book.

According to **Lao Tzu**, living is all about "spontaneity" which holds the key to stress management.

What is spontaneity?

According to Tao, spontaneity is "doing without over-doing"—which essentially means "doing without *consciously* anticipating the outcome."

In the universe, there is an all-controlling force that monitors everything. You breathe in oxygen and breathe out carbon dioxide. You eat and you eliminate. You grow, mature, and deteriorate. In nature, spontaneity is evident in the change of seasons. Spontaneity is the natural built-in mechanism in each living organism. Spontaneity creates balance and harmony, expressed in the relationship between *yin* and *yang* (the female and the male)

According to **Lao Tzu**, everyday something is dropped; therefore, less and less do you need to *force* things "to happen" until ultimately you arrive at "non-action." When nothing is done, nothing is left *undone*—this is the essence of "doing without doing." It may seem paradoxical, but there is so much truth about that statement; in Tao, "nothingness" is paradoxically *everything*. The wisdom is that when you are in the middle of nothing, you are actually in the presence of *all* things and *everything*.

The explanation is that everything originally came from nothingness, that is, before the Creation—the nothingness is the Creator. That also explains why Tao is beyond words, because words are finite and the Creator is infinite.

There is a Chinese idiom that says: "Push the boat with the current." It means the wisdom of availing an opportunity to move forward without exerting too much effort; or, figuratively, to make use of judicious guidance according to circumstances. It is the wisdom of choice to empty oneself and go with the flow of the current, instead of against it. "Non-doing" is an act of spontaneity and effortlessness in accomplishing things.

"Non-doing" also means "going against the stream, not by struggling against it, but by doing *nothing*—just standing still and letting the stream do all the work." It does not literally mean "doing nothing." It is the wisdom of taking perfect action without initiating the action.

The problem with people in the Western world is that they are so "action-oriented" or preoccupied with the "doing"—usually out of fear, worry, or doubt of the outcome—that they fail to understand the power of their thought (Never underestimate your mind power; it is often mind over matter). As a result, ironically enough, their "doing" may hinder the progress of their efforts, and hence creating a *reverse* result. That is to say, they are striving to force their desire through action into manifestation of their expected outcome; and, by doing so, they mess up what they are trying to do.

It is often the "doing" that becomes a stressor in real life.

However, that is not to say that action is unimportant. As a matter of fact, it is not your action that makes things happen; quite the contrary, it is your *intent* that creates the desire that generates the positive energy that propels the action to manifest the outcome.

Hence, the "doing" becomes "non-dong" because it is *effortless*. When doing something becomes effortless, the stress disappears, and you feel more relaxed. "Non-doing" is developing daily habits of not making "much ado about nothing" in everything. Remember, stress hinders progress.

Dealing with Life's Problems

Life is riddled with puzzlements. Don't strive to solve them—or even to understand them. Remember, many of your problems will resolve by themselves, if you would give them time.

Problems inevitably create stress and tension—often a strain on your emotions. Worry, stress and tension are negative emotions that will often make a bad situation worse.

Learn to control your emotions, instead of letting your emotions control you. When you find an inner calm within yourself, you will be able to take better control of your life and live by your choices rather than by your reactions. Above all, learn to manage your anger.

Life is always going to throw difficulties in your way; learn to take them in stride.

One of the most important life lessons is learning to let go. According to **Buddha**, attachment is the root cause of all human miseries, and hence the source of stress and distress in life.

Letting go is the readiness and willingness to let go of all attachments in life, including time.

Many of us think that time is precious, and wish that we had more than 24 hours a day. We no longer have the time to appreciate the beauty of nature, because we have become overwhelmed by our daily problems and the time needed to solve them. Indeed, many of us are forever time-stressed.

Attachment to time means the reluctance to live in the present moment. Unfortunately, the present moment is the only reality in life, and the only moment during which one can objectively validate one's past thoughts and future projections that continuously filter through one's subconscious mind, enticing it to form identities—which become the components of one's ego-self.

If you let go of your attachments, your burden in life will become less stressful. According to **Jesus**, the burden in life will never be too much for you:

> "Take my yoke upon you, and learn of me; for I am meek and lovely in heart; and ye shall find rest upon your souls. For my yoke is easy, and my burden is light." (**Matthew** 11: 29-30)

A yoke is not an instrument of torture—rather, a special device to lighten the burden.

Remember, your Creator will never give you too many problems in life that are beyond your capability to deal with them. Just remember that, and you will be free from undue stress of contemporary living. Without the stress, many of your *myasthenia gravis'* symptoms will gradually disappear.

EIGHT

RELAXATION TO BOOST IMMUNITY

Stress

Many autoimmune diseases can be attributed to stress; as a matter of fact, stress is one of the underlying causes of many human diseases and disorders.

Too much stress can disrupt your body's production of hormones and thus indirectly affecting your immunity with an impact on the level of T cells and antibodies. Chronic stress can considerably compromise the majority of your immune responses.

Given that stress is inevitable in contemporary living, your body's capability to respond to stress and then to return to normal functioning holds the key to maintaining good health. In other words, relaxation of the body and the mind is essential to controlling and managing your symptoms of *myasthenia gravis*.

Signs and Symptoms of Stress

Some typical signs and symptoms of a distressed body and mind include the following: aggression and anger;

breathing problems; eating disorders; excess sweating; fatigue; headache; indigestion; irritability; memory loss; muscle tension; and poor concentration.

Remember, stress or distress is one of the key factors contributing to aging and chronic diseases. Anxiety and depression—often the byproducts of stress—are often the precursors to such autoimmune diseases as diabetes and rheumatoid arthritis. By accelerating breathing, elevating blood pressure, and constricting blood flow, stress may be the culprit of heart diseases. Even cancer can be adversely affected by distressed emotions. It is, therefore, important to learn relaxation techniques to *de*-stress yourself.

Sleep

Sleep, which is one of the most basic human needs, is often ignored. Natural sleep is an immune system booster. Sleep is the best anti-stressor for your body and mind. Build up your body's stress-proof reserves by getting adequate sleep. Sleep, like diet and exercise, is important for your mind and body to function normally.

During sleep, many of your body's major organs and regulatory systems continue to work actively, and in fact some parts of your brain actually increase their activities dramatically, producing more of certain hormones.

An adult needs between 7½ to 9 hours of sleep per day, that is to say, an average of 8¼ hours. Sleep deprivation is a health hazard. According to the National Sleep Foundation, nearly 20 percent of drivers admitted to dozing off at the wheel. This attests not only to the danger of loss of sleep but also to the general sleep deprivation in the United States. As a matter of fact, two-thirds of Americans say they have less than eight hours of sleep a night.

We all know that sleep is important, and yet many of us

are willing to sacrifice sleep for other priorities in our lives. It is a myth that you can *adapt* yourself to getting *less* sleep so that you may have more waking time. If you think you can be a thief of time and outsmart Nature, think again! Your accumulated "sleep debt" will always have to be paid back somehow in the form of sleep disorders, which may aggravate *myasthenia gravis* symptoms.

Fatigue due to insufficient sleep will take its toll somehow and sometime. That is the reality! As a matter of fact, your immune system needs as much as 9½ hours of sleep in *total darkness* (so, turn off all lights even though you can sleep with some lights on) in order to recharge your immune system completely. Unfortunately, many of us seldom, if ever, get as many as 8 hours of sleep on average. As a matter of fact, some experts even contend that getting too much sleep is as bad as not getting enough sleep. The bottom line: Get an average of at least 7 to 8 hours of sleep to boost your immune system.

Don't get smart by trying to get by with *less* sleep!

What makes you sleep?

You are put to sleep by two processes: *sleep homeostat*, which tells you to go to bed after a certain amount of time awake, and to wake up after a certain amount of time of sleep; and *biological clock*, which is a daily cycle unique to each individual.

But your biological clock can *overcome* your sleep homeostat—unless your "sleep debt" is much too huge. Therefore, if you *force* yourself to stay awake, you may be able to actually *stay* awake but at the expense of making you more prone to future sleep disorders.

A dark sleep environment is essential to a *full* rest. Your body is not *completely* shut down until there is *complete* darkness, which is conducive to healthy sleep.

You are not healthy unless your sleep is healthy. Sleep

that requires medication is *never* healthy.

Do not take sedative drugs, such as *Restoril®* and *Ambien®*; they may affect the thinking of older people, as well as contribute to daytime fatigue.

Are you getting adequate sleep? Not getting adequate sleep of eight hours is often due to many factors: such as longer work hours; health problems, such as arthritis pain, ulcers, or headaches; nutritional deficiencies, such as inadequate calcium; and stress, causing anxiety, worry, or physical tension.

Obvious signs of sleep deprivation include: lack of concentration, impaired memory, loss of interest in exercise, and higher stress, among others.

The amount of sleep required for optimum immunity health is unique to each of us. Research studies demonstrate that there is a genetic basis for our individual sleep requirement. A good way to find out how much sleep you need is to go to bed at the same time each night, and find out what time you naturally wake up without an alarm.

It is also important to find out your best sleep cycle. If you wake up still feeling tied after a full night' sleep, move your bedtime earlier until you wake up, feeling refreshed. Let your body adjust to the new sleep cycle.

Points to remember about getting natural deep sleep:

Keep a *regular* bed and wake time, even on weekends and holidays, so as not to drastically upset your biological clock. This is an important factor in forming good sleep habits.

Create a bedtime ritual for yourself, if needed. Parents often give their sleep-resistant children a routine ritual before putting them to sleep. This strategy can also apply to grown-ups. You can meditate for 20 minutes, or read some Bible verses before retiring. Always maintain a relaxing daily routine prior to sleep, such as a relaxing bath, or a glass of hot drink.

Do not get into the habit of watching TV to make you doze off. Once the habit is formed, you may find it difficult to sleep *without* the TV. Avoid bad habit-forming.

Maintain an optimum sleep environment. Temperature affects your sleep, because your body temperature plays a pivotal part in the sleep process. Your body temperature changes according to your biological clock, which induces good sleep. Remember, your body temperature rises in the early evening, and gradually cools down throughout the night until around 4 o'clock in the morning.

Therefore, the temperature of the bedroom and that of your bed must be optimum to induce natural sleep, that is, a temperature in the range of 62°F (16° C) and 71° F (24° C); anything above or below that temperature range may cause restlessness that prevents good sleep.

Adjust the humidity of your sleep environment. A too-dry sleep environment may cause bronchial passages, leading to constant coughing, which interrupts deep sleep. To prevent dryness, place a bowl of water to humidify the bedroom environment, especially in winter with the heat on. On the other hand, a too-humid bedroom causes dampness, which may raise your stress hormone levels. To avoid dampness, you may want to have your bed linen made from natural fabrics to help absorb any perspiration as well as to allow your skin to breathe more freely.

Pay attention to the intensity and color of light in your sleep environment. If you are accustomed to or have acquired the habit of sleeping in a dark environment, then the intensity of light is critical to obtaining good sleep. Colors are also important to natural sleep. For example, blue and green colors are generally more relaxing, and thus more sleep promoting than red and yellow colors.

Therefore, the use of drapes or shades, and bedroom decor can also help you sleep better.

Avoid any stimulant, such as caffeine, nicotine, or alcohol during the day, or especially before bedtime, although you may have grown accustomed to the stimulant.

A firm and supportive mattress induces good natural sleep.

Do not nap too much during the day: a long afternoon nap may rob you of your night sleep.

Do not eat at least 3 hours before bedtime: a full stomach makes sleep more difficult. Eating increases your metabolic rate as well as your body temperature, which are critical factors in natural sleep. Body temperature dropping is conducive to good sleep. That explains why you should not eat at least three hours before going to bed. A high body temperature prevents you from falling asleep, not to mention the bloated feeling that may bother you if you eat too much before bedtime.

Generally, it is better to eat smaller meals than to eat one heavy meal with one or two light meals in between. Eating too much at any one meal stresses not just your digestive system but also your brain.

Avoid foods that may impair your sleep health. Eating cheese, for example, may give rise to nightmares because it contains tyramine, an ingredient in cheese that can elevate blood pressure. MSG (monosodium glutamate), a taste enhancer in most restaurant cuisines, may cause digestive upsets, heartburns, and headaches, which often interrupt natural sleep. Yellow tartrazine (E-102), often added to fizzy drinks, candies, and cookies, may also increase hyper-activity that may prevent you from falling asleep fast. In short, foods that damage your health may also impair your sleep health.

Get some natural light in the afternoon each day. That,

surprisingly, may help you sleep better at night.

Regular daily exercise may enhance the quality of your sleep at night. But do not exercise right *before* bedtime.

If you feel that you need more than 24 hours a day to get all your things done, you are not alone.

But do tell yourself that a refreshed sleep will help you get things done faster and more efficiently, and that sleep is just a way to recharge yourself. Do not overwork to deprive yourself of sleep; you must develop the no-rush mentality.

If you toss and turn in the bed because of inability to sleep, get up and do some pleasant things—like a breathing exercise or meditation. Even if you can't go back to sleep right away, you will at least get to relaxing yourself, and hopefully you will soon become drowsy again.

To treat insomnia, you may like to lightly wind a soft cotton bandage around your forehead, eyes, and temples to exert light pressure on your facial muscles to induce a relaxed sleep.

Research studies have shown that all living things sleep. A Swiss research study indicated that gold fish, having been deprived of sleep for an extended period of time, would stay still for a protracted period of time to make up for its sleep deprivation; and that also applied to cockroaches. In other words, sleep deprivation would only lead to an increased need for sleep later, and all animals need sleep and instinctively know how to sleep. Man is no exception: sleep health is the essence of his being, without which there is no self-healing. Therefore, healing an autoimmune disease requires natural good sleep.

Other Relaxation Techniques

Relaxation holds the key to managing stress. Relaxation reduces your body's response to the effects of stress.

Relaxation helps recovery and recuperation from your autoimmune disease. In addition to a night of good sleep, there are other relaxation techniques.

There are basically *four* other types of relaxation: passive relaxation, such as watching TV, going to a movie or a ballgame; active relaxation, such as dancing, exercising, and making love; creative relaxation, such as painting, reading, and writing; and deep relaxation, such as sleep, meditation, hypnosis, mind aerobics, color therapy, and mental attention.

Deep Relaxation

Deep relaxation slows your brain by calming your body, slowing the metabolism of your heart and respiration rates, lowering your blood acidity, and reducing your muscle tension, thereby making you more *conscious* of your surroundings. Deep relaxation has been shown to help reduce tension, headaches, as well as jaw, neck, and lower back pain.

Practice deep relaxation techniques:

- To relax your *face*, clench your jaws as tightly as possible, hold for five seconds, and release. Smile broadly, hold for five seconds, and then release. Raise your eyebrows, hold for five seconds, and release. Repeat as necessary.

- To relax your *fists*, clench and hold them for five seconds, and release. Stretch out your fingers and thumbs, hold for five seconds and release.

- To relax your *eyes*, close them tightly for five seconds, and then open them again. Keep your neck straight and your body in a straight line. Widen your eyes as much as possible. Keep your head still, look upwards, and hold for five seconds. Now, roll your eyes slowly to the right, and focus on something, and hold for five seconds. Keeping your head still, roll your eyes down, focus, and hold for five seconds. Now, roll your eyes to the left, still keeping your head still, focus and hold for five seconds. Roll your eyes upwards again, and repeat the process one more time in the other direction. Finish by closing your eyes, and relax your head and shoulders. (For more eye-relaxation exercises, go to **NINE**)

- To relax your *shoulders*, consciously lift them, feeling your muscles tense, hold for five seconds, and then release. Now pull your shoulders down, hold for five seconds, and then release.

- To relax your *neck*, till your head forward, feeling tension on the back of your neck, hold for five seconds, and then release. Till your head to the left, feeling tension on your neck, hold and release. Repeat for the right side.

- To relax your *legs*, point your toes away from your body, and tighten your thigh muscles by stretching them. Hold for five seconds and release. Now, bend your right foot at the ankle and tighten your calf muscle. Hold and release. Repeat for the left foot.

Deep relaxation exercises are especially good for *myasthenia gravis*, with muscle weakness.

Deep relaxation is a luxury in this day and age, especially when everything in your life is fast-paced and hectic. But there is more to life than measuring its speed. Stress and tension constrict energy in the nerves of your body. Deep relaxation consciously remits energy to different parts of your body—a precursor to any physical, mental, spiritual self-healing. In addition, deep relaxation and controlled breathing reduce anxiety, and can help you deal with the issue at hand with a more relaxed and open mind.

Meditation

For thousands of years, meditation has been practiced in the East as a discipline to attain tranquility and spirituality. The health benefits of meditation have been documented: increasing mental sharpness; lowering blood pressure; preventing heart disease; and reducing chronic pain.

Meditation is a proven mind-body therapy for body-mind relaxation.

The healing power of meditation lies in its capability to focus the mind solely on the very *present moment*, thereby removing memories of the past and worries of the future. Meditation helps you focus your mind on the present moment to the exclusion of past and future thoughts. The mind in its natural and perfect stillness relaxes completely.

In contemporary living, your mind is often riddled with thoughts of what you just did, what you will do, or should have done. Nearly all your thoughts, including your desires and fears, are based on either the past or the future. Your desires are no more than recollections of the past pleasures and hopes of repeating them in the future. Fears are also memories of past pain, and your efforts to avoid the pain in the future. All of these rambling thoughts in your subconscious mind indirectly affect your conscious mind, and hence your body and your eyes.

In the present, your mind is always preoccupied with the

past or the future, leaving little or no room for the present moment, which, ironically enough, is the *only* reality. The past was gone, and the future is unknown; only the present is "real." The present is a gift, and that is why it is called "present." But, unfortunately, most of us do not live in the present, not to mention appreciate it, because the present is interlaced with the past and the future. Meditation is about re-focusing the mind on the present moment, so as to put both the past and the future into perspective.

The mental focus of meditation is not quite the same as the mental concentration on solving a difficult math problem or while performing a complex mental task. Meditation is about focusing on something seemingly *insignificant* (such as your breathing) or *spontaneous* (such as eating and even driving) such that your mind can be conditioned to focusing on only the present moment. In this way, your mind concentration excludes all past and future thoughts, so as to give your mind a meaningful break. It is in this sublime mental state that you are capable of understanding the true nature of things, and their relativity to the meaning of life and existence. Meditation awakens you to what is real or what is *quasi* real.

How to meditate

Points to remember when you meditate:

Focus on an *object* as your focal point of concentration: your own breathing; looking at a candle flame; listening to a sound; watching your footsteps when you are walking; or just about *anything* that can easily draw you back to your meditation.

- Palming exercise is an excellent exercise not just for vision improvement, but also for deep meditation.

- During your meditation, if your mind wanders away (which is quite common), gently direct your mind to re-focus on the object of your concentration. You learn how to focus through your act of *noticing* that your mind has wandered off, as well as through your repetitive efforts of *returning* to your meditation.

- Meditation is all about focusing on the present moment. Make focusing a habit of relaxation not just for your eyes but also for your mind and body.

- Keep yourself in *full consciousness*: you must be fully aware of what is going on around you. That explains why in meditation (except in the walking meditation) you need to sit erect in order to keep your body in full consciousness. Do not lie down (or else you may fall asleep); do not slouch (this may not help you focus).

- Maintain a *consistent* position or posture with your thumb tip and forefinger tip of each hand touching very lightly, while the other fingers are either curled or extended out. A consistent posture and hand position will promote a *meditative mind* to help you practice your meditation techniques.

(For more information on meditation, go to **Appendix A**)

How to breathe right to meditate and to relax

Breathing is important in meditation because it is the focal point of the mind. In addition, breathing out is associated with "letting go" and "body detoxification"—essential components in relaxing the body and the mind.

In meditation, focus on your natural breath as it flows in and out. Notice how you inhale and exhale. You will begin to feel yourself becoming totally relaxed and soothed.

Practice *diaphragm breathing* and *alternate-nostril breathing.*

Diaphragm breathing (the complete breath)

Consciously change your breathing pattern. Use your diaphragm (the diaphragm muscle separating your chest from your abdomen) to breathe in and out. If you place one hand on your breastbone, feeling that it is raised, with the other hand above your waist, feeling the diaphragm muscle moving up and down, then you are practicing diaphragm breathing correctly. Deep breathing with your diaphragm gives you complete breath.

This is how you do diaphragm breathing:

- Sit comfortably.

- Begin your slow exhalation through your nose.

- Contract your abdomen to empty your lungs.

- Begin your slow inhalation and simultaneously make your belly bulge out slightly.

- Continuing your slow inhalation, now, slightly contract your abdomen and simultaneously lift your chest and hold.

- Continue your slow inhalation, and slowly raise your shoulders. This allows the air to enter fully into your lungs to attain the complete breath.

- Retain your breath with your shoulders slightly raised for a count of 5.

- Very slowly exhale the air. The upper chest deflates first, and then the abdomen relaxes in.

- Repeat the process.

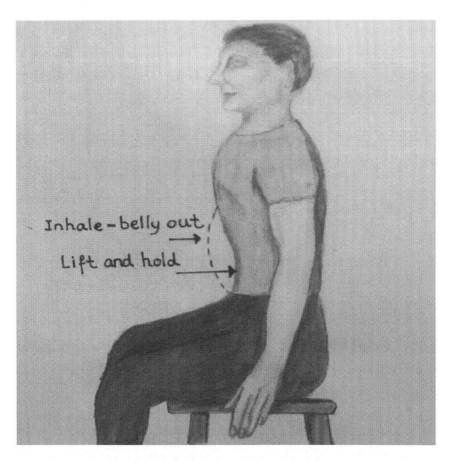

Learn to slowly prolong your breath, especially your exhalation. Relax your chest and diaphragm muscle, so that you can extend your exhalation, making your breathing out complete.

To prolong your exhalation, count "one-and-two-and-three" as you breathe in and breathe out. Make sure that they become balanced. Once you have mastered that, then try to make your breathing out a little longer than your breathing in.

Alternate-nostril breathing

Alternate-nostril breathing is a basic Yoga breathing exercise to balance the right side and the left side of your brain. Practice alternate-nostril breathing during meditation or as often as you require for body-mind relaxation. (For more details, go to **Appendix B**)

There are many meditation techniques. The easiest one is *awareness meditation*, which you can practice practically anywhere and anytime.

- Close your eyes.

- Be aware of your breath: notice *how* you breathe, your body's reactions to your breaths, such as your lungs and abdomen.

- Be aware of the flow of energy and blood throughout your body.

- Be aware of the surrounding, such as the sounds, the temperature, the odor, the lighting conditions, and the movements around you. Focus your attention on them, instead of on any thoughts that might drift into you mind.

- Do this for a few minutes per session.

You will soon experience perfect calmness, and your mind will become totally relaxed.

Mind Aerobics

Mind aerobics is a state-of-the-art sound technology, integrated into soothing music, to create positive lifestyle changes in listeners to help them overcome stress or achieve personal goals. Specifically, this amazing sound technology can actually put the human mind into different stages of deep relaxation, focused learning, enhanced memory, and overall wellbeing.

This technology is based on the scientific theory that in human beings certain electrical patterns in the brain correspond to different mental abilities and different mental states.

- In your waking consciousness, your *beta* brain waves provide you with concentration, alertness, and cognition. At its highest levels, *beta* waves may result in anxiety and disharmony.

- When you become relaxed, your *alpha* brain waves are in control, resulting in better concentration and more focused learning. In this mental state, your brain has the ability to learn, process, store, and recall large amounts of information quickly.

- If you become even more relaxed, such as when you are sleeping, your *theta* brain waves are conducive to increased memory and integrative experiences, which enable you to look deeply into your inner self: you see who you really are in relation to others and certain life situations. *Theta* brain waves not only increase your creativity, but also *de*-stress you.

- If you relax still further, your *delta* brain waves (the slowest of all brain waves) put you in a deep trance-like dreamless sleep while still making you mentally alert.

In addition to reducing stress and sharpening your mind, mind aerobics can increase longevity by suppressing *cortisol*, the age-accelerating hormone while increasing DHEA, the precursor of all hormones.

If you believe the "Mozart effects" can improve intelligence and enhance cognitive capabilities, then mind aerobics can certainly induce deep relaxation to reduce your stress and sharpen your mind.

Mind Concentration

Remember, the healing of any disease begins with the mind, and mind healing is always mind over matter. To initiate any meaningful change in your life or to begin self-healing, you must rely on your mind, specifically, your subconscious mind. Give your mind the tools to heal.

Again, how often we look at something without seeing it at all because our minds are not paying full attention to what we are looking at. When the mind is not paying full attention, the body becomes incapacitated; when the body becomes fully conscious, the mental capacity becomes enhanced and sharpened.

Body awareness is simply paying full attention to what your body is doing at that present moment. In other words, be conscious of what your body is doing when you are eating, walking, or doing anything.

Living in the present holds the key to relaxing the mind and hence the body.

Practice awareness whenever and wherever possible.

Walking is another opportunity for practicing body awareness. While walking, pay conscious attention to your breaths, the movement of your limbs, as well as the details of the environment. If you are listening to your music or talking on the cell phone while walking, you are depriving yourself of body awareness.

Eating and walking are the best times to practice daily body awareness and mind training for relaxation.

Body awareness has many benefits contributing not only to a healthy body and mind, but also to happiness in life:

- It increases the free flow of internal energy (*qi*), which carries oxygen and nutrients to nourish your body cells and tissues, and hence improving your overall mental and physical health.

- It sharpens mind power through concentration to initiate intentions.

- It creates the groundwork for mindfulness, which is focusing on what is happening around you, especially the people around you. Mindfulness leads to compassion, which is a quality that affords joy derived from the happiness of others.

- It prepares the mind for meditation, which ultimately holds the key to relaxation and clarity of mind.

- It promotes optimum breathing, which plays a pivotal role in enhancing mental relaxation and improving clear thinking.

Intense presence of the mind

To relax the mind and the body, intense presence of the mind is required. Try to do the following:

Close your eyes, and consciously wait for your *next* thought.

As you become more alert, anticipating the next thought, you will be surprised to find that it takes a while before your next thought actually arrives.

Why? Because your mind is in a state of intense presence, in which the mind is free of thoughts, and so the next thought does not come right away. By stilling the mind, you are relaxing your mind. When you are fully present, you are in a state of full alertness and relaxation because your mind is no longer immersed in thoughts of the past or their projections into the future.

The following are examples of intense presence of the mind:

For example, you can focus your mind on your daily chores, such as washing dishes. Pay full attention to the sound and feel of the water from the tap, the bubbles and scent of the detergent in the kitchen sink. If you do just that, instead of watching the television or listening to the radio, you will feel very relaxed after doing the dishes, and you will not look upon it as an unpleasant chore anymore. Try this tonight, and feel the difference in your mind.

For example, when you are waiting for the bus or the train, do not just let your mind wander. Instead, focus your concentration on, say, a building close by: trace the outline of the building with your eyes, and shift your eyes from looking at one window to another. In that way, you are training your mind to stay in the present moment, and thus stopping your compulsive mind from wandering off.

For example, you can focus your mind on an object, such as the cup you are holding in your hand. Say, while you were considering buying that cup from a store some time ago, you looked carefully at its shape, style, and design to decide if you wanted to buy it; but ever since you bought it, you have never looked closely at it again. Learn to re-focus your attention on the cup every time you are holding it in your hand; in that case, you are training your thinking mind to stop thinking, even though for just a brief moment. Look closely at the cup every time you are holding it in your hand.

Practice all of the above, or anything out of your own imagination, until concentration on the present moment becomes a habit and second nature to you. Focusing on the present moment works wonders on anxiety and stress.

Focusing the mind on the present moment is re-directing your concentrated attention on something *insignificant* or *irrelevant* that you are currently doing in order to stop your compulsive mid from thinking of past thoughts or projecting them into the future.

Healthy living focuses on the present moment through relaxed breathing and mind concentration.

NINE

OVERCOMING MUSCLE WEAKNESS

Muscle Weakness

Muscle weakness is one the major symptoms of *myasthenia gravis*. Muscle weakness, which can occur in any part of the body, may lead to progressive weakness and further deterioration due to lack of muscle use. In other words, the muscle weakness may go from bad to worse. This may result in difficulty in undertaking routine movements, setting off muscle wastage and nerve deterioration further down the road.

In *myasthenia gravis*, muscle strength is normal when resting. This has led many to believe that rest is the *only* option, but this is not true.

When I was diagnosed with *myasthenia gravis*, the doctor told me to rest whenever I complained about my muscle weakness. Many doctors are too willing to comply with the wishes of their patients. I found out that exercise holds the key to eliminating muscle weakness.

Research is clear on two points: oxygen deficiency (due to lack of exercise and incorrect breathing) decreases immune function; moderate amount of mild exercise increases immunity.

Oxygen plays a pivotal part in a healthy immune system. Nobel Prize winner **Otto Warburg** found the link between oxygen deficiency and the development of cancer cells. Oxygen plays a key role in your immune function because it provides ammunition for killer and natural killer T cells, as well as antioxidants.

Exercise enhances your oxygen intake and tunes up your metabolism. Both Yoga and Qi Gong conserve and generate your energy, and thus making you feel less fatigue. In addition, the rhythmic movements of these ancient Oriental exercises not only deepen your breath but also relax your muscles through the act of contracting and releasing; their postures further enhance the circulation of lymph, a fluid in your lymphatic system responsible for cleansing your immune system.

Use *soft-movement exercises,* such as Yoga or Qi Gong to overcome muscle weakness.

Yoga

Yoga health can have therapeutic effects on muscle weakness of *myasthenia gravis* through a series of mild and easy body movements in conjunction with deep breathing techniques to enhance muscle tone as well as to reduce any physical pain. Yoga exercise practice requires neither energy nor strength. Instead, through the gentle movements, the muscles are moved, worked, and toned, with a new flow of energy into the body from the natural movements, while the enhanced blood circulation also strengthens the weakening muscles. In addition, because Yoga health is holistic health, it also addresses the anxiety and fear issues of muscle weakness experienced by an individual with *myasthenia gravis.*

The bottom line: Although the muscle groups may be weak, they still need to be exercised: "use it or lose it" still applies to muscle weakness of *myasthenia gravis*.

Yoga health provides the most practical approach to attaining a high level of physical fitness, as evidenced in muscle strength and flexibility attained through Yoga exercises and Yoga postures.

Do not let the debilitating muscle weakness overwhelm you. Instead, overcome your muscle weakness with Yoga health.

Do the following basic Yoga exercises:

- Stand with your feet shoulder-width apart. Slowly raise and stretch out both hands in front of you.

- Notice your breath, and feel the stretch along your arms and your legs (which have to be firmly rooted onto the ground), as well as around your waist. Hold the stretch for 30 seconds.

- Slowly release your arms and place them by your sides.

- Slowly rotate your head sideways, and back and forth, to stretch your neck muscles.

- Repeat the process.

The next Yoga exercise not only helps you let go of all you negative energies but also promotes your full body circulation to prepare you for the day ahead. More importantly, it can improve your body posture, which is an essential component of natural healing.

- Stand with your feet apart (shoulder-width apart), and heels turned out.

- Slowly let your body drop in front of you, with your arms loosely hanging down.

- Inhale slowly as your body relaxes further down.

- Slowly drop your chin to your chest as you release your spine, one vertebra at a time. Do not lock your knees, while slowly exhaling.

- Notice your breath, as you release your spine, shoulders, arms, fingers, neck, face, jaw, and eyes.

- Slowly return your body to a standing position.

- Repeat the process.

This third Yoga exercise not only relaxes the body, including the mind and the eye, but also massages the internal organs, such as the liver, kidneys, and intestines. This relaxed Yoga posture exercise helps you let go of all your anxieties and fears about muscle weakness, and stimulate the neuromuscular system to muster more muscular strength.

- Stand with your feet shoulder-width apart, and heels slightly turned out.

- Interlock your fingers of both hands behind your back.

- Inhale slowly until your lungs are full.

- Slowly lift the center of your chest, open your shoulders back, and then pull your arms down, while slowly exhaling.

- Stand firmly with the back of your knees open.

- Notice your breath and how your chest is lifted and fully open, with your arms pulled back. Maintain this posture for at least one minute.

- Now, slowly release your arms, and let them rest by your sides.

- Repeat the process.

This Yoga exercise tones your arm muscles as well as stimulates the kidneys, the liver, and the intestines to enhance internal body detoxification. By expanding your lungs, it also relieves anxiety and fear.

Given that the postures of Yoga exercise are designed to strengthen, stretch, and tone muscles and ligaments, with emphasis on particular parts of the body, you can effectively target any body part with muscle weakness. Because Yoga involves both the breath and the mind, Yoga relaxes the whole being and reduces stress, which is the enemy of *myasthenia gravis*.

Qi Gong

Qi Gong is an ancient Chinese healing art that integrates mental practice and visualization (motor imagery) into exercises for posture, body movement, breathing, and energy work. The word "qi" means "life force" or "internal vital energy of the body," and "gong" means "accomplishment" or "skill" that is cultivated through steady practice. Qi Gong is also called "the new yoga."

The gentle, rhythmic exercises of Qi Gong mirror the movements of nature, especially the fluidity of water. In conjunction with its unique and simple breathing techniques, the ancient Qi Gong exercise is uniquely suited to strengthening not only the immune system but also the body muscles, thereby increasing the body's innate healing abilities.

Unlike some Yoga routines, the Qi Gong "flow" routines can be learned very quickly, and therefore ideal for muscle weaknesses related to *myasthenia gravis*.

Research studies have attested to the promotion of "relaxation response" by Qi Gong exercise—a phase in which your body relaxes and rebuilds, thereby instrumental in producing chemical messengers to reduce any high level of adrenal hormone to stimulate your immune system.

Therefore, to maintain some physical strength, to enhance neurological signals, and to regain some muscle strength, the mental practice of Qi Gong with motor imagery is ideal for strengthening muscles. Motor imagery, which is picturing, sensing and feeling doing a physical action, may be instrumental in stimulating the neuromuscular system to muster more muscular strength to perform the exercise routine. According to scientific data, Qi Gong exercises can help re-wire the nervous system, creating new neurons and synapses, attesting to the benefits of the mental practice, which is a major component of the Qi Gong exercise.

Get some Qi Gong lessons from your local Qi Gong master, or watch Qi Gong videos, showing how to move your body in a state of flow, while returning your mind to the present moment to create balance and harmony for internal healing.

Walking

Walking is also a perfect activity for those who are not well enough to pursue a more vigorous exercise. Walking is the closest to perfect exercise for those with *myasthenia gravis*, especially with muscle weakness in the legs. Studies showed that walking may have other substantial health benefits, including reducing the risk of coronary heart disease and stroke, lowering blood pressure, reducing high cholesterol and improving good cholesterol level.

Brisk is best. Brisk walking is walking without overexertion; in other words, you should be able to hold a conversation while you are walking. Of course, the intensity of walking varies according to your age and your own muscle strength. Even a 10-minute brisk walk can increase your muscle fitness, provided that it is *brisk* enough.

It should be stressed that you should also be *mindful* when you are walking. Mindfulness can add a meaningful dimension to your walking: it not only accelerates your body-mind interaction, which is critical to any healing process, but also enhances your awareness of *how* your mind may affect your body in matters of health. Do not approach walking as if you are merely performing a function of your body. Paying detailed attention to *how* you walk *is* mindful walking. Do not talk on the cell phone while you are walking.

Exercises to Balance and Stretch

Body balance

Due to your muscle weakness, especially in your legs,

you may find it difficult to maintain your body balance, and therefore more prone to falling.

Find your own *focal point* by focusing your eyes on an object. Practice your body balance by slightly raising one foot, either right or left, in the following positions:

- Both hands on your hips

- Both hands at your sides

- Both hands outstretched sideways

- Both hands raised above your head in a "V" position

Strengthening legs for balance, equilibrium, and mobility

- Sit on a chair, and relax, with feet apart, and hands on your sides.

- Stand up a little, with legs bent, and hands on your sides, and HOLD at a count of five.

- Next, stand up a little more, with legs still slightly bent, and hands on your sides, and HOLD at a count of five.

- Now, stand up straight and tall, and HOLD at a count of five.

- Reverse and repeat the process until you sit down on the chair.

Enhancing body balance and flexibility

- Stand tall, your feet slightly apart, with your arms stretched out sideways for body balance.

- Slowly bend your right knee, and cross your right foot in front of and to the outside of your left foot, touching your right toes to the floor.

- With your right knee still bent, slowly and gently SWING your right leg from the front position to behind your left leg, touching your right toes to the floor. Use your stretched out arms to balance if necessary.

- Repeat the activity using your left foot.

Stretching

Stretching has substantial benefits for muscle weakness: it increases your mobility range, your muscle flexibility, your energy level, your blood circulation, and your protection against injury should you happen to fall.

Wake-up stretches

Stretch your limbs before you get out of bed every morning.

Extend your arms over your head and extend your legs as far as possible until you feel the stretch in the tips of your fingers and toes. Meanwhile, inhale deeply through your nose. Then breathe out deeply and slowly while drawing your arms down along the side your body with your palms facing up. You will feel full relaxation in your legs. Repeat the stretches several times to energize as well as to relax your body.

Do a single or double knee hug. Start by bringing your knee into your chest. Massage your hip joint by moving your leg in circles in both directions. Repeat with the other knee. Finally, hug both knees into your chest, raising your nose to your knees as much as possible. Now, relax your body and let your knees fall gently down to either side. Repeat the whole process several times for stretch and relaxation.

Yoga and Qi Gong are exercises that also stretch your body and limbs to promote flexibility.

TEN

OVERCOMING VISION PROBLEMS

Weak Eye Muscles

Given that *myasthenia gravis* is a neuromuscular disorder, the muscles and the nerves that control vision are often adversely affected.

The muscles that create movement and vision are normally under your conscious control. However, the *involuntary* muscles (such as the muscles of your heart and many other organs, including your eyes) are beyond your conscious control. In *myasthenia gravis*, weakness occurs because the nerves that activate your eye muscles fail to stimulate them as a result of your immune cells (which normally attack foreign invaders) targeting and attacking your body's own healthy cells—known as an autoimmune response.

Double Vision

If your eyes are misaligned and concurrently look at two different targets, two non-matching images will be sent to your brain. When your brain accepts and uses two non-

133

matching images at the same time, double vision inevitably occurs—one of the hallmarks of *myasthenia gravis*.

In an attempt to avoid double vision, your brain will eventually disregard one of the mismatching images. That is, your brain will ignore one eye (called suppression).

Due to your brain's capability to suppress one eye, your double vision can temporarily go away, or its effect becomes less pronounced. However, the problem is still there. Specifically, you may gradually lose vision of one eye—the one that your brain is ignoring; in addition, you also lose normal depth perception and stereo vision.

Ocular myasthenia gravis is a type of *myasthenia gravis* that affects only the eyes and eyelid movement. The hallmark of *ocular myasthenia gravis* is eye muscle weakness that increases during activity and improves after rest.

Common ocular myasthenia gravis symptoms include:

- Drooping of one or both eyelids (ptosis)

- Blurred vision due to weakness of the muscles that control eye movements

- Double vision (diplopia) due to weakness of the muscles that control eye movements

Ocular myasthenia gravis symptoms may vary in severity in different individuals.

Eye Relaxation

Eye relaxation is important to how the eye muscles may function optimally.

Eye relaxation begins with the mind *first*, not the eye.

The mind must be *completely* relaxed before it can relax the body—and the eye, which is only one of the organs of the body.

Relax the Body to Relax the Eye

Practicing Qi Gong, Tai Chi, and Yoga can relax the body, the mind, and hence the eye because these exercises focus on "soft" movements of the body.

Western-style exercises, on the other hand, focus more on building physical strength and muscles rather than on relaxing the muscles for total body relaxation.

Self-Massage to Relax the eye

Self-massage the eye for relaxation to increase blood circulation, to create a sense of ease about seeing, and to enhance eye awareness for better vision.

Facial and eye massage

- Breathe deeply and slowly.

- Rub both hands to generate warmth.

- Massage your jaw with your hands moving in small circles, from the chin outward along your jawbone up to the front of and behind your ears.

- Then, move your hands over the bridge of your nose, and then massage outward along your cheekbones until you reach your temples and your ears.

- Then, starting from the bridge of your nose, massage along your eyebrows, moving above, below, and along the brow. Use your thumbs to press against the grooves slightly below your eyebrow ridge close to the bridge of your nose.

- Gently squeeze your eyeball with your fingers.

- Finally, use long, firm, strokes to massage your forehead from the left to the right, and then from the right to the left.

Throughout your facial and eye self-massage, look for sore spots, especially in the eyebrow area. Massage them with slightly harder and stronger circular movements.

Rub the eye

- Apply and press the heel of your left palm and the heel of your right palm against your left eye and right eye, respectively.

- With gentle pressure, rub with a twisting movement your left eye with your left palm and your right eye with your right palm.

- Meanwhile, contract and relax your eyelid muscles.

Acupressure for eye massage and eye relaxation

Apply pressure and massage from your fingers to stimulate all the acupressure/acupuncture points around your eyes.

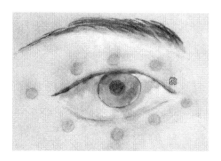

Eye Exercises to Relax the Eye

Regular eye relaxation

To overcome eyestrain, which causes weak eye muscles, you need regular eye relaxation for optimum vision health:

- Consciously breathe in and breathe out through your nose to bring more oxygen to your eyes, as well as to reduce any stress on your vision. Learn diaphragm breathing and alternate-nostril breathing (Go to **Appendix B**).

- Loosen your shoulders and keep them down to allow as much oxygen as possible to fill up your lungs as you breathe in through your nose.

- Push out as much as possible the carbon dioxide from the bottom of your lungs, feeling your stomach and chest flatten out gradually as you breathe out through your nostrils.

- It is important that you do not *force* yourself to *inhale*; instead, wait for your natural impulse to breathe in again. Repeat the process until your breathing becomes a natural rhythm.

- Concentrate your mind on only breathing and nothing else.

- Meanwhile, let your eyelids droop until they gently close. Your eyes should be *unfocused* and your eye muscles *relaxed*. Slightly open your mouth, while dropping your jaw.

- Continue breathing for a few minutes with your eyes closed.

- Now, open your eyes. When you re-open your eyes, do not focus immediately on anything in particular.

- Blink your eyes repeatedly to soothe and moisturize your eyes. If possible, induce self-yawning.

- Smile broadly and hold for five seconds to remove any tension you might be holding in your eyes.

Practice eye relaxation as often as required, especially when you feel eyestrain with *myasthenia gravis*, for better vision health.

Palming to relax the eye

This unique eye-relaxation exercise uses your healing hands to direct energy to your eyes, as well as to rest your optic nerve and relax your entire nervous system.

Unlike sleep, which is unconscious and passive relaxation, eye-palming is conscious and active relaxation. Therefore, eye-palming is one of the best exercises for eye relaxation. Practice palming at least for 10 to 30 minutes per session for three or more sessions daily to completely relax your eyes. Even at work, you can palm your eyes for 2 minutes, if possible, to relieve your eyestrain from the computer.

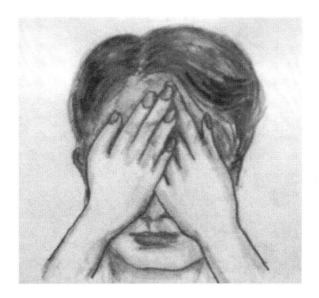

- Sit comfortably with your elbows resting on a table in front of you—preferably in a darkened room, such as a bathroom without any window.

- Rub your palms together to generate some warmth.

- Place your palms over your eyes, without touching them, while resting them on the boney ridge surrounding your eyes with the heels of your hands on your cheekbones. Your eyes should be *gently* closed.

- Relax your mind, and breathe deeply through your nose, not your mouth. The slower your breathing is, the more relaxed your mind becomes.

- Feel your abdomen and back expand and contract as you inhale and exhale, respectively.

- Visualize complete darkness to relax your mind.

- Feel your neck and shoulders expand and contract as your deep and slow breathing continues.

- Visualize every part of your body—hands, fingers, toes, knees, and thighs—expand and contract with your inhalation and exhalation.

Practice eye-palming whenever you feel fatigue in your eyes. It is impossible to palm for too long or for too much; some palm for hours to reap the benefits of both relaxation and meditation. If you feel any resistance to palming, it may probably be due to your subconscious mind's resistance to relaxation. If you become more relaxed, you will see *complete blackness.* However, it is all right if you do not see complete blackness; just continue with your daily palming exercise.

Remember, we are living in a stressful world, and many of us simply cannot relax, even if we very much would like to. Attesting to the inability to relax, many of us easily and often stare without blinking—and, worse, without being aware of it. As a result, our vision slowly and gradually deteriorates over the years.

The "8" eye exercise for relaxation and flexibility

Do the following "8" eye exercise as often as required to relax your eye muscles as well to increase their flexibility.

- Sit comfortably in a relaxed posture.

- Consciously breathe in and breathe out through your nose until you attain a natural rhythm.

- Imagine the figure "8" in the distance.

- Let your eyes *trace* along the imaginary figure without moving your head.

- First, trace it in one direction, and then in the opposite direction.

You can modify the exercise by imagining other alphabets and figures. The objective of this exercise, in addition to promoting relaxation and flexibility, is to train your eyes to consciously *shift* when focusing on an object in the distance, instead of eye-fixation or staring.

The Taoist squeeze-and-open eye exercise for blood circulation to relax the eye

This ancient Chinese exercise developed by Taoist monks thousands of years ago increases blood circulation to the eyes, prevents watery eyes, and alkalizes the eyes to detoxify the liver. It removes eyestrain and soothes eye-muscle tension.

- Inhale slowly, while squeezing your eyes tightly for 10 seconds.

- Then, slowly exhale your breath, making the sh-h-h-h-h sound, while opening your eyes wide.

- Repeat as many times and as often as required to

cleanse the eyes and the liver.

Learn how to blink

If you do not blink frequently enough, you will not be able to see well. It is just that simple. Blinking has many vision benefits:

- It overcomes the harmful habit of staring.

- It relaxes the eye.

- It cleanses and massages the eye.

- It improves nearsightedness.

Learn how to blink, not *squint*. The former relaxes the eye, while the latter stresses the eye because it uses undue force to close and open the eye.

Practice the following exercise as frequently as needed to make blinking second nature to you:

- Breathe deeply.

- Close and open your eyes. The blink has to be *soft*, not hard, and it must be *complete*. Imagine using your eyelashes to cause your eyes to close and open. Practice this several times until you master it. You may even count while you blink to make sure you do not blink too fast.

- Close your right eye, and cover it with your right hand.

- Blink your left eye. If the blink is soft, and not forced, your right hand over your right eye will not feel any movement. It is important that your blinking has to be soft and effortless.

- Repeat the process with the other eye.

Always remember to blink several times before you look at something in close vision and in distant vision. Habit forming is important.

Yawning to cleanse and relax the eye

Yawning is a natural way to relax the body and the mind, as well as to cleanse the eye and the liver.

- Practice yawning *deliberately* with wide-open jaws, while expelling sounds through your mouth. If possible, induce tears from your eyes.

- After a few yawns, close your eyes, and relax.

- Now, with eyes closed, use your nose to draw the figure "8" vertically, horizontally, and diagonally (nose painting).

With practice, you can yawn *anytime* and *anywhere*, even when you are not tired.

Stretching eye muscles for relaxation

Master the eye-muscle stretching exercise to relieve eye tension and maintain eye relaxation.

- Sit comfortably, taking a few deep breaths.

- Stretch your eyes upward as far as they can go without straining them.

- Hold your breath. Stretch your eyes downward as you exhale.

- Repeat this up and down movements of your eyes a few times.

- Stretch your eyes by moving them around in circles, but without straining them, as you breathe in and breathe out.

Perform this exercise anytime and anywhere, such as waiting for the bus, standing in line, or walking.

Softening vision for relaxation

The elephant-swing exercise

Practice this basic Qi Gong exercise—the elephant swing—to enhance circulation, relaxation, peripheral vision, soft vision, and integration of vision. This is an excellent all-in-one exercise for overall vision improvement.

- Stand with your feet parallel, about 10 inches apart.

- Gently close your eyes.

- Shake your arms and legs, and roll your neck sideways, back and forth until they become soft and relaxed.

- Still your mind, and breathe naturally.

- Now, open your eyes, and look at what is in front of you. Remember not to stare.

- Slowly swing your body to the left and then to the right by shifting your weight from one foot to the other and lifting the heel of each foot as you turn in a swaying motion. Let your arms hang loosely, and let your head move with your body, not by itself. The movement should be soft, natural, and relaxed, without any strain.

- Notice that the surrounding seems to "move" in the opposite direction. Let your eyes "shift" naturally without fixing on anything.

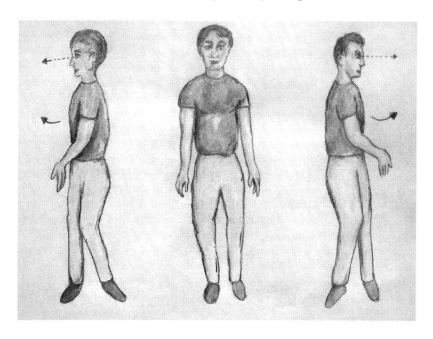

Practice this elephant-swing exercise as often as you can to soften your vision and to improve your overall vision health.

Strengthening Vision

The macula in the center of the retina is responsible for detailed vision. Overuse of the central vision leads to weakening of the macula, resulting in much loss of detailed vision. This is not uncommon for those suffering from *myasthenia gravis*.

Increasing peripheral vision will decrease the use of central vision, and hence instrumental in protecting the macula and enhancing detailed vision, which is critical to good vision.

- Cut small black rectangular cards in different sizes (2"x 2"; 2"x3"; 2"x5") from construction paper. Tape the card to the top of the bridge of your nose, covering part of both eyes.

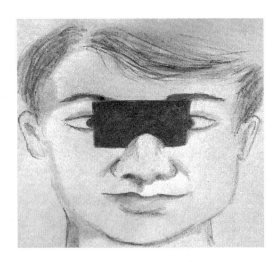

- Sit or stand, and look through the smallest black

rectangular card in front of your eyes, while turning your head from side to side.

- Notice that your surrounding seems to be "moving" in the opposite direction.

- Stop turning your head, and close your eyes for a minute or two. Now, visualize the previous "moving surrounding" in your mind's eye.

- Open your eyes again, and move or wave your hands on both sides of your ears. Notice your moving hands, which are now stimulating your peripheral cells.

- Stop waving your hands, and close your eyes. Now, visualize the movement of your hands in your mind's eye.

- Repeat the above with the mid-size and then the large-size black rectangular cards.

By partially covering the eyes, your mind enables your eyes to pay more attention to what is on both sides, and hence stimulates your peripheral vision. After each exercise, you will see that your vision has "expanded" and has become "broadened." By strengthening your peripheral vision, you indirectly reduce your use of central vision, and hence protecting your macula from deterioration and degeneration.

The bottom line: Regular eye exercises are critical to maintaining vision health, especially for those with *myasthenia gravis*. It is important to have the patience and perseverance to do these eye exercises on a daily basis. You may not see the results immediately, but the benefits are long-term.

ELEVEN

THE JOURNEY OF
DISCOVERY AND RECOVERY

If, unfortunately, you or your loved one has developed *myasthenia gravis* or an autoimmune disease, there is no need to despair. Your Creator may have given you or your loved one the disease as an opportunity to turn life around for the better. Look upon the autoimmune disease as an opportunity for personal growth and development, as a journey of self-discovery, or simply as a blessing in disguise. Remember, life is always a bed of roses but with some thorns.

Embark on your journey of discovery and recovery. This may not be an easy journey, but begin your first step anyway.

> "The journey of a thousand miles begins with the first step." **Lao Tzu**

Taking the first step, however, may be easier said than done. In order to take the first step towards self-discovery and health recovery, you must, accept the fact that you are afflicted with an autoimmune disease. Irrespective of your current health conditions, you have to continue to live your life, so make the most of it, and do the best you can to make a comeback from your setback.

Acceptance paves the way to transformation. Very often, it takes a human tragedy or health crisis to change human perceptions of self and life. Like myself, you may learn a valuable lesson from your *myasthenia gravis*. It may teach you how to overcome despair, how to function within your limitation, and, above all, how to fight back.

Once you begin your first step on the road to recovery, you understand that the journey requires you to make some changes in your life. In order to bring about the necessary changes, you need to empower yourself with knowledge and information to change what is undesirable, and to turn what is deemed desirable into a reality.

Knowledge empowerment often helps you develop an inquiring mindset—a lifelong tool for health and wellness.

Given that the human mind naturally reacts and responds when it focuses on a thought prompted by a question, your inquiring mindset makes you ask many thinking questions about health and wellness—especially regarding all the hypes from the media, the medical community, as well as from the food and drug industries.

An inquiring mind is a mind of wisdom: always being aware of the need to see total perspective of everything in all its relationships; always knowing the most important things in life (health is certainly one of them) and understanding how best to go about getting them. In the inquiring mental process, you learn how to become a healthier person despite getting your *myasthenia gravis* (which may be a blessing in disguise) with the right thinking resulting in the right conduct towards your body, mind, and spirit for holistic recovery.

Being knowledgeable, you may also develop positive mentality that gives you self-belief: that you can do what is necessary to cope with your disease symptoms.

You *must* change your thinking in order to change your action to change your life.

"What the mind of man can conceive and believe, it can achieve." **Napoleon Hill**

Changes can change your self-belief. It is important that you believe you can bring about recovery no matter what. There are, however, two obstacles that may dampen your self-belief: comparing and looking back. Don't compare you current health with that prior to your immune disease, or with that of other healthy individuals; don't look back with regret over the wrong things you had done in your life, leading to your autoimmunity. Comparing and looking back would negatively undermine your self-belief.

With self-belief, you begin to see the potentials of your recovery, and all the possibilities available to you.

Sir William Osler, the Canadian physician, the father of modern medicine, once said: "The good physician treats the disease; the great physician treats the patient who has the disease." So, if your physician is treating only your disease symptoms, you should be the one to treat *yourself* who have the disease. In the process, you may discover that a good autoimmune diet along with other dietary supplements can effectively reduce your autoimmune reaction by controlling or slowing down the over-production of antibodies, which attack your immune system, resulting in your autoimmune disease.

"The only way to keep your health is to eat what you don't want, drink what you don't like, and do what you'd rather not." **Mark Twain**

Your discovery of foods as medicine may also change your diet completely: you begin to eat organic whole foods to temper your autoimmune response that may have come from your digestive system. Strange as it may seem, nearly 30 millions of Americans are suffering from autoimmune disorders, there is not yet a recognized autoimmune diet that focuses on combating autoimmunity through nutrition. In treating yourself who has the disease, you may discover your own autoimmune diet through food addition and elimination. Your food allergies may also be the culprit.

To take good care of your digestive health to improve your immune system, you would have to cleanse it every now and then. You begin with a one-day water or fruit detox, and then pursue a longer fast of one to two weeks. Remember, after the third day, you would not feel any physical hunger or food craving; so a longer fast is more psychological than physical. A more complete fast detoxifies your whole body, eliminating all toxins that may have wrecked your immune system, causing autoimmunity.

A regular one-day fast is necessary for maintenance of optimum digestive health. In addition, regular fasting is also weight maintenance. Remember, excess body weight exerts undue pressure on weak muscles and joints.

"Take care of your body. It's the only place you have to live." **Jim Rohn**

Take care of your body by exercising. Don't let your muscle weakness be a stumbling block on your way to physical recovery. Don't let muscle atrophy happen due to lack of use. Yoga, Qi Gong, Tai Chi, or any flexibility exercise not only relaxes your body and mind, but also strengthens and tones up your muscles.

On the journey of discovery and recovery, do not look back with regret over what you should or should not have done over the years. Let bygones be bygones. Always look ahead, and visualize a healthy you in your mind's eye.

On the journey, you may encounter remissions and relapses; it is only natural. Do not look for a miracle cure, because there is none. Instead, look for self-healing from within yourself, and not from the outside. Any autoimmune disease is a complex disorder involving the entire body system; accordingly, searching for a limited treatment, such as the use of medications, to cure the disease is only self-delusional. The only possible and probable cure is a holistic approach to overall health and wellness of the body, the mind, and the spirit. As a matter of fact, healing comes from the mind—the right mindset to believe in the capability to heal; the right mindset to empower oneself with knowledge and tenacity to heal; and the right mindset to overcome all obstacles encountered in the healing process. In other words, use your mind power to give your body the opportunity to heal itself.

Follow the wisdom of **Dr. William Bates**, the founder of natural vision. According to his profound wisdom on vision: do not try to see clearly *now*; you will see clearly when your vision improves, but not *before* that. That is to say, do not try to see clearly with vision aids, such as eyeglasses or contact lenses, because they only temporarily improve your vision but impairing your long-term vision health.

By the same token, do not strive to suppress the symptoms of your autoimmune disease with dangerous steroid medications; the symptoms will gradually disappear when the overall physical, mental, and spiritual health improve over time. According to **Hippocrates**, the father of medicine, nature cannot be rushed. So, be patient, and your healing is on the way.

Given that the symptoms of an autoimmune disease can be severe, refraining from taking medications can be a difficult choice—a choice that nobody can make for you.

Marcel Proust, the celebrated French writer, once said: "To believe in medicine would be the height of folly, if not to believe in it were not a grater folly still." His statement seems to have put many of us in a catch-22 situation.

Indeed, the reliability of pharmaceutical drugs reflects more of a statistical reality than an accurate prediction. On the other hand, any blanket recommendation to cure or reduce the many symptoms of autoimmune diseases, including *myasthenia gravis*, may be too good to be true. Just remember that the human immune system has too much variability and idiosyncrasy to successfully map out a blueprint to tackle its autoimmunity. In short, what works for me or anyone else, may not work for you. Therefore, the wisdom is to acquire as much knowledge as possible about the disorder, its causes, and the strategies to deal with its symptoms. With mental intent, you may be able to cooperate with your compromised immune system, leading to a better prognosis. Only you know what it is like to live every day with your autoimmune disease. Only you know that even a small relapse or an infection can trigger off the onset of yet another autoimmune episode. Avoid any trigger, such as stress, food allergy, or environmental toxin. Do as much as you can; you cannot be doing too much. Just do it!

Good luck!

Stephen Lau

APPENDIX A

MEDITATION

Meditation is thinking about one thing at a time. Simple as it may seem, this requires practice and discipline. According to **St. Theresa of Avila**, the mind is like an unbridled horse wandering where it will, and your role is to train the horse, and gently and lovingly bring it back to the right course.

Meditation is training your mental attention to sharpen your awareness of what is going on in your mind. Once you see clearly what is going on in the present moment, you can then choose to ignore or to act upon what you are seeing through your mind.

For thousands of years, people have been transforming their minds and hence their lives through this simple mind training. Meditation can be done in silence and stillness, through sounds, or even body movements—as long as the focal point is mental attention and awareness of the present moment.

Whatever that gets your attention will control and dominate you. In other words, your habitual responses precondition your mind. Therefore, the primary purpose of meditation is to refocus and pay careful attention to your experiences and responses as they go through your mind; you just observe, without judging them. The objective of observing without any judgment is to eliminate as much as possible any automatic and reflexive response that leads to the pre-conditioning of the mind. Simply put, don't jump to conclusion *yet*; get all the details *first*, and then evaluate them *objectively*.

The Meditation Process

Meditation is a simple process that can be practiced by every one of us. The meditation process involves:

- Quieting the mind: observing thoughts and feelings with no judgment

- Controlling the mind: taming a wandering or an overactive mind

The meditation process can last from 10 minutes or so to more than an hour. Just let it happen *naturally*.

Meditation Basics

To meditate, you must get into the right frame of mind; that is, you must learn some meditation basics in order to know *how* to meditate effectively:

- You must be in a quiet environment conducive to meditation.

- Your body must be comfortable and still, and very relaxed.

- Your breathing must be right: inhale and exhale softly and slowly, preferably in a rhythm.

- Your mind must be focused, staying in the present moment, as much as possible.

- You must not expect anything to happen during the

meditation session. You must always practice with consistency and persistence.

How to Meditate

Find a quiet place where you can remain undisturbed for 10 to 30 minutes. To set the environment for meditation, you may want to have some scent from flowers, or even some soothing music (meditation MP3) to enhance your senses. Of course, you can meditate without them; it is just an option, not a requirement.

Find time to practice meditation. Regularity holds the key to success in meditation. Do not meditate only when you feel like it. Find some quiet time to yourself everyday. The ideal time to meditate is before retiring to bed; in that way, your mind can review what has happened during the day—what you have said and done—and let go of everything. After all, meditation is about letting go of the past and future thoughts.

Correct posture is also important. Firstly, your body must be erect: this induces correct breathing, which can bring all your internal energies into a state of harmony. Therefore, do not lean back on anything. If you find that your neck is too weak and your spine cannot support your body, then rest your back on a hard surface initially; but the ultimate goal is to sit erect without your back touching anything.

You can sit cross-legged on the floor. Alternatively, you can sit comfortably on a chair (not a sofa), with your thighs at right angles to your spine, your hands on your thighs, your feet resting firmly on the floor, and your shoulders relaxed. In short, just sit "tall" and erect.

Begin meditation with your breathing. Your breathing is an indicator of your stress level: if you are unduly stressed, your breathing becomes thick and gasping. Breathing right is your conscious control of stress. When you feel stressed, consciously change your breathing pace to undo the stress.

Gently close your eyes, or you can fix your eyes on an object, such as a candle.

As you begin your meditation, you will find that your first thought does not come to your mind right away. When it finally comes, do not dismiss it. Instead, consciously focus on your breathing. That thought will then slowly disappear. After a while, another thought or the same thought may come up to your mind. Again, do not consciously dismiss it; refocus on your breathing. With more practice, you will find that within a 10-minute time frame, fewer and fewer thoughts will crop up in your mind because your mind has stayed in the present moment for a longer period. The fewer thoughts you have, the more relaxed you become.

Then, one day, you suddenly find that you have stepped into a different world with total tranquility and clarity of mind—even though it lasts but a very brief moment. That out-of-the-world sensation is nondescript. Once you have attained that inexplicable and transformative state of mind, you will want to continue practicing meditation everyday. But don't expect that transcendental state will come any time soon; the more you expect it, the longer it will take you to attain that state of mind. Just consistently and patiently practice meditation everyday with no expectation other than relaxing your body and mind.

Meditation is life-changing: it may change *how* you look at yourself and the world around you, especially now that you have an autoimmune disease.

APPENDIX B

ALTERNATE NOSTRIL BREATHING

Alternate-nostril breathing is a basic Yoga breathing exercise to balance the right side and the left side of your brain.

The left side of your brain governs the right side of your body, including your speech and logical thinking, while the right side of your brain governs the left side of your body, including your creativity and intuition. Achieving balance and harmony between the two sides of your brain is critical to mind healing for deep relaxation. You can balance your mental energy from the right and the left side of the brain through practicing alternate-nostril breathing any time during meditation or in any mind-relaxation session. Practice alternate-nostril breathing everyday for mental balance and relaxation.

How to Practice

- Place your thumb and ring finger lightly on your right and your left nostrils, respectively, with your index and middle fingers resting lightly on your forehead between your eyebrows.

- Exhale deeply through BOTH nostrils.

- Press your thumb against the RIGHT nostril to CLOSE it.

- Breathe in through your LEFT nostril. Count 8.

- CLOSE your LEFT nostril by pressing down your ring finger. Now, BOTH nostrils are closed. Retain the air, and count 4.

- OPEN your RIGHT nostril, and breathe out. Count 8.

- With the LEFT nostril still CLOSED, breathe in through the RIGHT nostril. Count 8.

- CLOSE the RIGHT nostril. Now, BOTH nostrils are closed. Retain the air, and count 4.

- OPEN the LEFT nostril, and breathe out with the RIGHT nostril still closed. Count 8.

- With the RIGHT nostril closed, you have breathed out through the LEFT nostril; you have now completed one round of the breathing exercise.

- Begin the second round by breathing in through the LEFT nostril, and repeat the above.

Practice your alternate-nostril breathing to create acute awareness and concentration, as well as to enhance internal body balance.

APPENDIX C

AWARENESS WALKING

Walking is one of the best exercises for the immune system. However, to reap the full benefits of walking, the walk must be brisk, with full awareness and deep concentration of the mind. Very often, we are so caught up with our destination that we put our feet into automatic pilot, while our minds drift from one thought to another. To stop our rambling thoughts, we must train our minds to concentrate through awareness while we are walking briskly.

Awareness walking requires you to pay full attention to what you are doing, to notice the movement of your limbs, the shifting of your body weight as you move your right and left foot. Awareness walking gives you an opportunity to quiet your mind, to practice subliminal messages, to enhance your mental concentration.

How to Walk with Awareness

For example, you can choose the first two verses from the famous **Psalm 23**: **"The Lord is my Shepherd. I shall not want."** Repeat each syllable in your mind with each foot as you walk step by step, one step at a time. Always begin with your right foot, and then followed by your left foot; continue your steps following each syllable with the corresponding right or left foot:

"The Lord is my She-pherd. I shall not want"
  R   L R L R L   R L R L

You always begin the first word with the right foot. So, if you have to begin the first word with the left foot instead, then you know that you have messed up somewhere; in other words, you mind must have wandered off. When that happens, start all over again with your right foot first, followed by your left foot. You may be very surprised that within a 10-to-20-minute walk you might have messed up the sequence and coordination several times, because your mind did not concentrate enough.

You can slightly adapt your favorite Biblical verses, such as **"Trust the Lord with all your heart and don't depend on your own understanding. Remember the Lord in all you do and He will give you success."** (**Proverbs** 3: 5-6), and turn them into subliminal messages, such as the following:

"I trust the Lord with all my heart. I de-pend on His

R L R   L   R   L R   L R L R   L R

grace for-e-ver. I re-mem-ber the Lord in all I do and

L   R L R L R L R L   R L R L R L

He will give me suc-cess."

R   L   R   L R   L

You can also create your own subliminal messages to practice awareness walking: **"I am healthy, strong, and in good spirit."**

Don't talk on the cell phone while you are walking. Instead, avail yourself the walking opportunity to sharpen your awareness, still your mind, and reinforce it with positive subliminal messages. Don't just exercise your body; also exercise your *mind* at the same time!

APPENDIX D

ACID AND ALKALINE BALANCE

Dr. Deepak Chopra, M.D., bestselling author, founder of the Chopra Center for Wellbeing, says: "If you don't take care of your health today, you will be forced to take care of your illness tomorrow."

Take care of your health today with acid-and-alkaline balance in your diet. A balanced acid-alkaline level increases your energy and vitality, neutralizes excess acids in your body, removes accumulated toxins in your blood, strengthens your weakened immune system and organ systems, destroys harmful microorganisms, and balances the pH in your body. In short, an optimum acid-alkaline balance holds the key to a healthy immune system that may work wonders on your autoimmune disease.

If you have insomnia, mood swings, chronic fatigue, aches and pain, dull skin, brittle hair and nails, difficulty in concentration, and other health issues, you do not have a balanced acid-alkaline level in your body.

Optimize your body's acid-and-alkaline level with your diet. Remember, some acid-forming foods may become alkaline if the acids are properly metabolized by the body. The goal is to attain balance. An optimum environment for cell replication and regeneration holds the key to a healthy immune system

Here is a list of common foods with their acid and alkaline levels for general reference:

Acid-Forming Foods	Alkaline-Forming Foods
rice bran	seaweed
dried fish	ginger
egg yolk	kidney beans
oatmeal	shitake mushrooms
brown rice	spinach
tuna	soybeans
chicken	bananas
pearl barley	chestnuts
oysters	carrots
salmon	mushrooms
buckwheat	strawberries
scallops	potatoes
pork	cabbage
peanuts	radishes, squash
beef	sweet potatoes
cheese	turnips
whole barley	orange juice
shrimp	apples
peas	egg white
beer	coffee, tea
bread	cucumber
butter	onions
asparagus	string beans
(acid level of foods in descending order)	(alkaline level of foods in descending order)

APPENDIX E

AN ANTI-INFLAMMATION DIET

Inflammation is a natural immune response to injury, toxins, allergy or infection. Because 70 percent of your immune system cells are located on the lining of your digestive tract, your immune response is greatly affected by the foods you ingest, especially foods that may cause inflammation.

The main causes of inflammation are as follows:

- Injury (a natural process of repairing injured cells or tissues)

- Allergy (the immune system overreacting to a harmless substance, such as a natural food, or potentially harmful substance, such as a synthetic chemical)

- Toxicity (cellular injury due to overexposure to toxic agents or chemicals in the environment, in processed foods, and in pharmaceutical drugs, among others)

- Nutritional imbalance (a deficiency or an excess of proteins, fats, carbohydrates, vitamins and minerals causing hormone disturbances, leading to a compromised immune system)

- Infection, such as a yeast, fungus, or bacteria attack

- Emotional trauma (increase of adrenaline and cortisol stress hormones due to excess or chronic stress)

Have a moderately low-calorie diet with emphasis on weight control. Foods that are high in calories are linked to higher amounts of inflammation, and the greater amount of fat tissue you have, especially around your midsection, the more inflammation you are going to have.

Most fresh fruits and vegetables are anti-inflammatory. Those red, yellow, or orange ones are particularly loaded with antioxidants, such as carotenoids, vitamin C, and quercetin. However, if you are sensitive to food allergies, avoid all "nightshade vegetables" that include eggplant, tomatoes, and potatoes because they contain a chemical called *solanine* that may trigger an inflammatory response in some individuals who have food allergies. Eggs, dairy products, and wheat are also associated with food allergies in some individuals.

Eat high-fiber whole grains, seeds and nuts to reduce levels of C-reactive protein.

Avoid all highly processed cereals, sweets, fruit juice, white breads and pasta that increase blood-sugar levels that may trigger the release of insulin and pro-inflammatory chemicals in your body.

Cook with anti-inflammatory herbs and spices, such as ginger, cayenne, clove, feverfew, nutmeg, oregano, and rosemary. Avoid charred or over-grilled foods.

Drink anti-inflammatory beverages, including white, green, and black tea (they contain antioxidant polyphenols), and red wine (but no more than 2 drinks per day).

Dark chocolate is also part of an anti-inflammatory diet.

Anti-inflammation is disease prevention and treatment because inflammation touches every aspect of human health.

ABOUT STEPHEN LAU

About Stephen Lau:
http://www.stephencmlau.com

Books by Stephen Lau:
http://www.booksbystephenlau.com

Stephen Lau's Related Sites:

http://www.wisdominliving.com
http://www.health-and-wisdom-tips.com
http://www.daily-tao-wisdom.com
http://www.chinesenaturalhealing.com

Made in the USA
Columbia, SC
08 March 2021